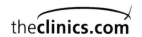
theclinics.com

INFECTIOUS DISEASE CLINICS OF NORTH AMERICA

Infectious Disease Emergencies

GUEST EDITORS
David A. Talan, MD
Gregory J. Moran, MD
Fredrick M. Abrahamian, DO

CONSULTING EDITOR
Robert C. Moellering, Jr, MD

March 2008 • Volume 22 • Number 1

SAUNDERS

An Imprint of Elsevier, Inc.
PHILADELPHIA   LONDON   TORONTO   MONTREAL   SYDNEY   TOKYO

W.B. SAUNDERS COMPANY
A Division of Elsevier Inc.

Elsevier, Inc., 1600 John F. Kennedy Blvd., Suite 1800, Philadelphia, PA 19103-2899.

http://www.theclinics.com

INFECTIOUS DISEASE CLINICS	**Volume 22, Number 1**
OF NORTH AMERICA	**ISSN 0891-5520**
March 2008	**ISBN-10: 1-4160-5085-X**
Editor: Barbara Cohen-Kligerman	**ISBN-13: 978-1-4160-5085-8**

The ideas and opinions expressed in *Infectious Disease Clinics of North America* do not necessarily reflect those of the Publisher. The Publisher does not assume any responsibility for any injury and/or damage to persons or property arising out of or related to any use of the material contained in this periodical. The reader is advised to check the appropriate medical literature and the product information currently provided by the manufacturer of each drug to be administered to verify the dosage, the method and duration of administration, or contraindications. It is the responsibility of the treating physician or other health care professional, relying on independent experience and knowledge of the patient, to determine drug dosages and the best treatment for the patient. Mention of any product in this issue should not be construed as endorsement by the contributors, editors, or the Publisher of the product or manufacturers' claims.

Infectious Disease Clinics of North America (ISSN 0891-5520) is published in March, June, September, and December (For Post Office use only: volume 20 issue 4 of 4) by Elsevier Inc., 360 Park Avenue South, New York, NY 10010-1710. Business and Editorial Offices: 1600 John F. Kennedy Blvd., Suite 1800, Philadelphia, PA 19103-2899. Customer Service Office: 6277 Sea Harbor Drive, Orlando, FL 32887-4800. Periodicals postage paid at New York, NY and additional mailing offices. Subscription prices are $202.00 per year for US individuals, $339.00 per year for US institutions, $101.00 per year for US students, $238.00 per year for Canadian individuals, $410.00 per year for Canadian institutions, $267.00 per year for international individuals, $410.00 per year for international institutions, and $131.00 per year for Canadian and foreign students. To receive student rate, orders must be accompanied by name of affiliated institution, date of term, and the *signature* of program/residency coordinator on institution letterhead. Orders will be billed at individual rate until proof of status is received. Foreign air speed delivery is included in all *Clinics* subscription prices. All prices are subject to change without notice. **POSTMASTER**: Send address changes to *Infectious Disease Clinics of North America*, Elsevier Journals Customer Service, 6277 Sea Harbor Drive, Orlando, FL 32887-4800. **Customer Service: 1-800-654-2452 (US). From outside of the US, call 1-407-563-6020. Fax: 1-407-363-9661. E-mail: JournalsCustomerService-usa@elsevier.com.**

Infectious Disease Clinics of North America is also published in Spanish by Editorial Inter-Médica, Junin 917, 1er A 1113, Buenos Aires, Argentina.

Reprints. For copies of 100 or more, of articles in this publication, please contact the Commercial Reprints Department, Elsevier Inc., 360 Park Avenue South, New York, New York 10010-1710. Tel. (212) 633-3813, Fax: (212) 462-1935, email: reprints@elsevier.com.

Infectious Disease Clinics of North America is covered in *Index Medicus, Current Contents/Clinical Medicine, Science Citation Alert, SCISEARCH,* and *Research Alert.*

Printed in the United States of America.

GUEST EDITORS

DAVID A. TALAN, MD, FACEP, FAAEM, FIDSA, Professor of Medicine, David Geffen School of Medicine at the University of California Los Angeles, Los Angeles; Faculty, Department of Medicine, Division of Infectious Diseases; and Chairman, Department of Emergency Medicine, Olive View–University of California Los Angeles Medical Center, Sylmar, California

GREGORY J. MORAN, MD, FACEP, FAAEM, Professor of Medicine, David Geffen School of Medicine at the University of California Los Angeles, Los Angeles; Faculty, Department of Medicine, Division of Infectious Diseases; and Director of Research, Department of Emergency Medicine, Olive View–University of California Los Angeles Medical Center, Sylmar, California

FREDRICK M. ABRAHAMIAN, DO, FACEP, Associate Professor of Medicine, David Geffen School of Medicine at the University of California Los Angeles, Los Angeles; and Director of Education, Department of Emergency Medicine, Olive View–University of California Los Angeles Medical Center, Sylmar, California

CONTRIBUTORS

FREDRICK M. ABRAHAMIAN, DO, FACEP, Associate Professor of Medicine, David Geffen School of Medicine at the University of California Los Angeles, Los Angeles; and Director of Education, Department of Emergency Medicine, Olive View–University of California Los Angeles Medical Center, Sylmar, California

MICHAEL T. FITCH, MD, PhD, FACEP, FAAEM, Assistant Professor and Neurosciences Program Faculty Member, Department of Emergency Medicine, Wake Forest University School of Medicine, Winston-Salem, North Carolina

GREGORY J. MORAN, MD, FACEP, FAAEM, Professor of Medicine, David Geffen School of Medicine at the University of California Los Angeles, Los Angeles; Faculty, Department of Medicine, Division of Infectious Diseases; and Director of Research, Department of Emergency Medicine, Olive View–University of California Los Angeles Medical Center, Sylmar, California

DAVID A. TALAN, MD, FACEP, FAAEM, FIDSA, Professor of Medicine, David Geffen School of Medicine at the University of California Los Angeles, Los Angeles; Faculty, Department of Medicine, Division of Infectious Diseases; and Chairman, Department of Emergency Medicine, Olive View–University of California Los Angeles Medical Center, Sylmar, California

CONTENTS

examination findings to identify patients at risk for these infections, and central nervous system (CNS) imaging and lumbar puncture (LP) may be needed to further evaluate for these diagnoses. The diagnosis of bacterial meningitis can be challenging, as patients often lack some of the characteristic findings of this disease with presentations that overlap with more common disorders seen in the emergency department. This article addresses considerations in clinical evaluation, need for CNS imaging before LP, interpretation of cerebrospinal fluid results, standards for and effects of timely antibiotic administration, and recommendations for specific antimicrobial therapy and corticosteroids.

FORTHCOMING ISSUES

RECENT ISSUES

ELSEVIER
SAUNDERS

INFECTIOUS
DISEASE CLINICS
OF NORTH AMERICA

Infect Dis Clin N Am 22 (2008) ix–xi

Preface

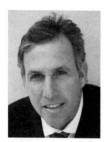
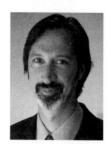
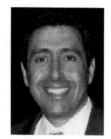

David A. Talan,
MD, FACEP, FAAEM, FIDSA

Gregory J. Moran,
MD, FACEP, FAAEM
Guest Editors

Fredrick M. Abrahamian,
DO, FACEP

This issue of *Infectious Diseases Clinics of North America* addresses infectious disease emergencies from the perspective of the emergency physician in the emergency department (ED). In this regard, we hope that it will be helpful to the infectious diseases consultant to the emergency physician. One might question how this perspective is different from that of an infectious diseases specialist consulting in any other setting. Two of the guest editors of this issue practice as both emergency and infectious diseases specialists, and, for almost two decades, have considered the interface of these disciplines and the uniqueness of infectious diseases as practiced on the front line of clinical medicine.

Time-dependent emergencies impact both diagnostic and treatment strategies. In the ED, the cause of the infection and antimicrobial susceptibility of the pathogen are usually unknown. At one time, the concept of withholding antimicrobial treatment until there was some degree of certainty about the infectious etiology dominated approaches to even acute infections such as suspected bacterial meningitis and sepsis. EDs were viewed as triage areas, and it was believed that parenteral antimicrobial therapy was most appropriately begun upon hospital admission and only after complete evaluation by the patient's admitting physician or an infectious diseases specialist.

Several factors probably led to greater prioritization of evaluations and empiric therapy in the ED. These included the establishment and development of the specialty of Emergency Medicine, facilitation of more rapid and accurate evaluation with improved diagnostic imaging modalities, such as spiral computed tomographic scanning and bedside ultrasonography, increased recognition of the relationship of time to appropriate therapy to improved outcomes, medical–legal pressures, and prolonged ED stays of patients awaiting hospital beds, including intensive care unit admission.

In addition, many infections previously thought to require prolonged inpatient treatment with parenteral antibiotics were found to be amenable to outpatient treatment, including community-acquired pneumonia and acute pyelonephritis. The introduction of long-acting parenteral antimicrobials, specifically ceftriaxone, and highly active and bioavailable oral antibiotics, such as fluoroquinolones, further facilitated ED outpatient disposition options. Since hospitalization dominated other costs, economic pressures in medicine focused more research on ED risk-stratification and outpatient treatment, which further increased the importance of ED care.

To an increasing extent, important infectious disease etiologic and epidemiologic investigations have been conducted through multicenter ED-based research. The sheer volume of cases through EDs allow larger studies of infections that are infrequent in other settings (eg, dog, cat, and human bite infections), and rapid recognition of emerging syndromes (eg, community-associated methicillin-resistant *Staphylococcus aureus* skin and soft tissue infections).

Whereas infectious diseases specialists consider antibiotic prophylaxis for opportunistic infections in immunocompromised hosts, emergency specialists routinely deliberate about prophylaxis in patients sustaining wounds, whether due to natural (eg, laceration and bite wounds) or iatrogenic trauma (eg, chest tubes and incision and drainage of an abscess). Decisions are made about the prevention of bacterial infection of a contaminated wound and other infectious complications, such as tetanus and rabies.

Most recently, major randomized controlled trials in the area of sepsis have led to new standards for early ED recognition and resuscitation. Management of this essential infectious disease emergency has expanded to include not only selection of appropriate antibiotics, but also initiation of therapeutic modalities considered outside of the traditional infectious diseases realm, such as hemodynamic optimization, source identification and control, and novel pharmacologic approaches including recombinant human activated protein C and supplemental corticosteroids.

Rapid and specific tests to identify occult infections that could only be identified no sooner than the next day by standard cultures may be around the corner, and their introduction will place even greater importance on the ED as a site for infectious diseases management. The ED will be the gateway for recognition and care of patients affected by natural and terrorism-related infectious disease epidemics. Infectious diseases specialists will need to work with ED staff to make plans to address ED surge capacity and coordination of diagnostic, infection control, and treatment strategies.

Finally, we hope that through these writings we can help bridge the gap between the specialties of emergency medicine and infectious diseases. Sometimes an infectious disease specialist acts as a "Monday morning quarterback," unfamiliar with the limitations imposed by evaluation and treatment decisions based on one brief encounter. Infections that appear full-blown later had to be evolving at some point earlier. A danger exists in a specialist's perspective in that the chance of serious infection being present among patients seen in infectious diseases consultation is many times greater than among undifferentiated ED patients. Clinical judgment must be used to avoid an unnecessary, extensive work-up and overtreatment for every febrile ED patient. With that said, much can be learned from the lessons only made obvious through tincture-of-time and careful subsequent evaluation and follow-up. More two-way communication between emergency and infectious disease physicians will enhance the knowledge of both types of specialists. It is with these insights that we hope to present our perspective through a review of infectious diseases emergencies.

David A. Talan, MD, FACEP, FAAEM, FIDSA
Department of Emergency Medicine
Olive View–UCLA Medical Center
14445 Olive View Drive
North Annex
Sylmar, CA 91342-1438, USA

E-mail address: dtalan@ucla.edu

Gregory J. Moran, MD, FACEP, FAAEM
Department of Emergency Medicine
Olive View–UCLA Medical Center
14445 Olive View Drive
North Annex
Sylmar, CA 91342-1438, USA

E-mail address: gmoran@ucla.edu

Fredrick M. Abrahamian, DO, FACEP
Department of Emergency Medicine
Olive View–UCLA Medical Center
14445 Olive View Drive
North Annex
Sylmar, CA 91342-1438, USA

E-mail address: fmasjc@ucla.edu

ELSEVIER
SAUNDERS

INFECTIOUS
DISEASE CLINICS
OF NORTH AMERICA

Infect Dis Clin N Am 22 (2008) 1–31

Severe Sepsis and Septic Shock in the Emergency Department

David A. Talan, MD, FACEP, FAAEM, FIDSA[a,b,c,*],
Gregory J. Moran, MD, FACEP, FAAEM[a,b,c],
Fredrick M. Abrahamian, DO, FACEP[a,b]

[a]David Geffen School of Medicine at University of California Los Angeles,
Los Angeles, CA, USA
[b]Department of Medicine, Division of Infectious Diseases, Olive View-University
of California Los Angeles Medical Center, 14445 Olive View Drive,
North Annex, Sylmar, CA 91342-1438, USA
[c]Department of Emergency Medicine, Olive View-University of California
Los Angeles Medical Center, Sylmar, CA, USA

Increased attention has focused recently on the acute management of severe sepsis and septic shock, conditions that represent the end-stage systemic deterioration of overwhelming infection. Clinical trials have identified new therapies and management approaches that, when applied early, appear to reduce mortality. Practice guidelines have been advanced by critical care societies, such as the Surviving Sepsis Campaign [1], and many of the proposed interventions involve therapies other than antimicrobials directed at hemodynamic resuscitation or addressing adverse effects of the inflammatory cascade. The infectious disease professional organizations have published practice guidelines that focus on antimicrobial management of clinical conditions such as pneumonia, urinary tract infections, and skin and soft-tissue infections, but have not published guidelines that primarily address severe sepsis or septic shock. As it has been estimated that approximately 458,200 sepsis cases annually in the United States (or 61% of sepsis presentations) are first encountered in the emergency department (ED) [2–4], infectious diseases specialists may not routinely engage in the initial diagnosis and management of these patients. Recently, ED-based sepsis management guidelines have also been published [5]. Although many EDs are now adopting treatment protocols for sepsis that are based on published treatment

* Corresponding author. Department of Emergency Medicine, Olive View–UCLA Medical Center, 14445 Olive View Drive, North Annex, Sylmar, CA 91342-1438.
E-mail address: dtalan@ucla.edu (D.A. Talan).

0891-5520/08/$ - see front matter © 2008 Elsevier Inc. All rights reserved.
doi:10.1016/j.idc.2007.09.005
id.theclinics.com

guidelines, initial enthusiasm for and extrapolation of many of these novel approaches have to some degree outstripped the appropriate confidence associated with the existing data from clinical trials. Recent research calls many of the initial recommendations into question, and validation trials of some of these approaches are ongoing. Given that patients with possible sepsis are frequently identified through the ED, the initial evaluation and treatment considerations of sepsis in this setting are reviewed.

Definitions

Sepsis is a term whose meaning has become confused over the years, as its traditional common-use meaning of a very ill, infected patient was redefined in an attempt to standardize its definition, especially for the purpose of establishing enrollment criteria for clinical trials [6]. More recently, the definition of sepsis has been modified back toward the more serious condition that clinicians typically associate with the term [7].

In 1992, an American College of Chest Physicians and Society of Critical Care Medicine consensus conference defined sepsis as the presence or presumed presence of an infection accompanied by evidence of a systemic response, called the *systemic inflammatory response syndrome* (SIRS). SIRS was defined as the presence of two or more of the following: (1) temperature above 38° or below 36°C; (2) heart rate above 90 beats/min; (3) respiratory rate above 20 breaths/min (or $PaCO_2$ <32 Torr); and (4) white blood cell (WBC) count greater than 12,000/mm^3 or less than 4000/mm^3, or greater than 10% immature band forms. It is important to recognize that this definition of sepsis would apply to many individuals with benign and self-resolving infectious syndromes, and some with non–infection-related conditions. From the standpoint of an emergency physician faced with a full range of patient presentations, these criteria are too nonspecific for the diagnosis of severe infection, whereas the predictive value of these criteria is naturally higher among the select group of patients seen in infectious diseases consultation. The issuance of this definition has unfortunately caused some to inappropriately conclude that all ED patients with SIRS criteria need to have extensive laboratory evaluation beyond basic clinical assessment or require hospital admission and administration of broad-spectrum intravenous antibiotics [8].

The consensus conference definition of *severe* sepsis was the presence of sepsis based on SIRS criteria and one or more sepsis-related organ dysfunction(s). Organ dysfunction can be defined as evidence of acute lung injury; renal failure; coagulation abnormalities; thrombocytopenia; altered mental status; renal, liver, or cardiac failure; hypoperfusion with lactic acidosis; and hypotension (fluid unresponsive). Of course, organ failures may be pre-existing or due to conditions other than sepsis. *Septic shock* was defined as the presence of sepsis and fluid unresponsive hypotension (ie, systolic blood pressure of <90 mm Hg), mean arterial pressure (MAP) <65 mm Hg (in adults), or a 40-mm Hg drop in systolic blood pressure compared with baseline unresponsive to a 20- to 40-mL/kg crystalloid fluid challenge (or requiring inotropes of vasopressors), along with perfusion abnormalities. Note that, by these definitions, septic shock is a subset of severe sepsis.

More recent investigations have determined that SIRS criteria for sepsis alone have no additional associated mortality compared with infection without SIRS, whereas organ dysfunctions (ie, severe sepsis) and refractory hypotension (ie, septic shock) are associated with worse prognoses than those found in patients with infection without these conditions [9,10]. In 2003, the North American and European Intensive Care Societies proposed a revised sepsis definition [7]. The new definition requires *some* of the many clinical and laboratory findings and, although still nonspecific, in general reflects a greater degree of abnormalities than SIRS (Box 1). Thus, the definition of sepsis has shifted back toward its common usage to reflect severe sepsis and septic shock.

As the pivotal clinical trials have enrolled patients who meet criteria for previous definitions of severe sepsis and septic shock, and to avoid confusion associated with the term "sepsis," this article refers to severe sepsis/septic shock together. *Bacteremia* is not considered synonymous with sepsis because *bacteremia* is often transient and asymptomatic, and also because viable bacteria in the blood are only found in about 50% of cases of severe sepsis and septic shock, whereas 20% to 30% of patients will have no microbial etiology identified from any source [12].

Clinical evaluation and laboratory testing

To diagnose severe sepsis/septic shock as early as possible, it is necessary to recognize historical, clinical, and laboratory findings that are indicative of infection, organ dysfunction, and global tissue hypoxia. Studies of the diagnostic utility of various laboratory tests, either alone or in combination, in addition to clinical findings amongst the broad-based ED population do not exist. The recommended laboratory studies and findings to detect severe sepsis/septic shock derive mainly from definitions of severe sepsis/septic shock and enrollment criteria of the pivotal clinical trials that are discussed below. A full discussion of the clinical diagnosis of severe sepsis/septic shock is beyond the scope of this article.

Certain laboratory abnormalities are among the criteria for sepsis (see Box 1), and therefore, various tests are recommended when an infection and multiple organ failure are suspected. These include a complete blood cell count (CBC) with the differential, standard chemistry panel, including bicarbonate, creatinine, liver enzymes, lactate, and coagulation studies. Clinicians have traditionally relied on the CBC—specifically, leukocytosis, neutrophilia, and bandemia (ie, premature granulocytes)—as indicators of both the presence of a bacterial etiology and as a measure of the severity of illness. However, these indicators have poor accuracy and thus cannot be used alone to either exclude or confirm the diagnosis of bacterial infection

Box 1. Diagnostic criteria for sepsis

*Infection[a] (documented or suspected) and some
of the following:*

General variables
    Fever (core temperature >38.3°C [101.0°F])
    Hypothermia (core temperature <36°C [96.8°F])
    Heart rate (>90 beats/min or >2 standard deviation
      above the normal value for age)
    Tachypnea (respiratory rate >20 breaths/min)
    Altered mental status
    Significant edema or positive fluid balance (>20 mL/kg
      during 24 h)
    Hyperglycemia (plasma glucose >120 mg/dL or 7.7 mmol/L)
      in the absence of diabetes
Inflammatory variables
    Leukocytosis (WBC count >12,000/mm^3)
    Leukopenia (WBC count <4000/mm^3)
    Normal WBC count with greater than 10%
      immature forms
    Plasma C-reactive protein greater than 2 SD above the normal
      value
    Plasma procalcitonin greater than 2 SD above the normal
      value
Hemodynamic variables
    Arterial hypotension (SBP <90 mm Hg, MAP <70,
      or an SBP decrease >40 mm Hg in adults or >2 SD
      below normal for age)
    SvO$_2$ > 70%[b]
    Cardiac index >3.5 L/min/mm^2
Organ dysfunction variables
    Arterial hypoxemia (PaO2/FIO2 <300)
    Acute oliguria (urine output <0.5 mL/kg/h or 45 mmol/L
      for at least 2 h)
    Creatinine increase greater than 0.5 mg/dL
    Coagulation abnormalities (INR >1.5 or aPTT >60 s)
    Ileus (absent bowel sounds)
    Thrombocytopenia (platelet count <100,000/μL)
    Hyperbilirubinemia (plasma total bilirubin >4 mg/dL
      or 70 mmol/L)

Tissue perfusion variables
  Hyperlactatemia (>2 mmol/L)
  Decreased capillary refill or mottling

Abbreviations: aPTT, activated partial thromboplastin time; INR, international normalized ratio; MAP, mean arterial blood pressure; SBP, systolic blood pressure; SD, standard deviation; SvO$_2$, mixed venous oxygen saturation; WBC, white blood cell.
  [a] Infection defined as a pathologic process induced by a microorganism.
  [b] SvO$_2$ can be low (<70%) in early sepsis, signifying inadequate oxygen delivery and global hypoperfusion. ScvO$_2$ (central venous oxygen saturation) has been used as a surrogate of SvO$_2$ [11].
  From Levy MM, Fink MP, Marshall JC, et al. 2001 SCCM/ESICM/ACCP/ATS/SIS International Sepsis Definitions Conference. Intensive Care Med 2003;29(4): 530–8; with permission.

[13–18]. Also, although extreme abnormality of the total WBC count and band proportion have been associated with sepsis-related mortality, they have a minor independent contribution among many other prognostic variables [19]. Again, when applied to the broad range of ED patients, their predictive accuracy for severe sepsis/septic shock is low. For example, in the derivation of the Pneumonia Severity Index, the total WBC count was not found to be an independent predictor of 30-day mortality among patients evaluated for community-acquired pneumonia, which is the most common site of infection in severe sepsis/septic shock [20].

Some laboratories report abnormal neutrophil morphology such as Döhle's bodies, toxic granulation, and vacuoles that are associated with the presence of bacterial infection [13]. Overwhelming severe sepsis can also be associated with leukopenia and neutropenia. Initial measurement of hemoglobin and hematocrit will commonly reveal hemoconcentration because of significant hypovolemia, and fluid resuscitation is expected to decrease red blood cell concentration. Since a hematocrit of less than 30% is a specific criterion for transfusion in resuscitation protocols, to be discussed below [11], repeat evaluations are recommended.

Thrombocytopenia, which frequently heralds the onset of disseminated intravascular coagulation, is an independent predictor of multiple organ failure and poor outcome [21]. In the Recombinant Human Activated Protein C Worldwide Evaluation in Severe Sepsis (PROWESS) study of 1690 patients with severe sepsis, a baseline elevated D-dimer and prolonged prothrombin time were observed in 99.7% and 93.4% of patients, respectively [22,23]. If severe sepsis/septic shock is suspected, platelet count and prothrombin time should be measured, with activated partial thromboplastin time, D-dimer, and fibrin degradation products and fibrinogen tested if there is evidence of disseminated intravascular coagulation.

Lactic acid levels are increasingly being employed to screen for global tissue hypoxia, as hyperlactatemia, along with SIRS criteria and suspected infection, was an enrollment criterion in one pivotal trial, to be discussed below [11]. A standard chemistry panel that reveals acidosis may represent the presence of lactic acidosis, and this may be an early clue to the existence of otherwise occult severe sepsis. Of note, hyperlactatemia is not always accompanied by a low bicarbonate level and/or elevated anion gap, and thus, a lactate level should be considered if severe sepsis is suspected [24,25]. Elevated lactate among ED patients admitted to the hospital with infection and upward trends in lactate levels are associated with poor prognosis and may be used to guide response to therapy [26–29]. Arterial lactate correlates well with mixed venous (pulmonary artery) and central venous lactate levels [30,31]. However, peripheral venous lactate should be interpreted cautiously owing to its inadequate agreement with arterial lactate measurements. The likelihood of arterial hyperlactatemia is reduced considerably by a normal peripheral venous lactate, but is only slightly increased if the peripheral venous lactate is increased [32]. Therefore, although a normal peripheral venous lactate helps exclude the presence of severe sepsis/septic shock, an arterial or central venous sample should be sent if a peripheral venous lactate is elevated.

More than 80 biological markers of sepsis—for example, C-reactive protein (CRP), interleukin 6 (IL-6), procalcitonin, protein C—have been investigated both for their diagnostic and prognostic capabilities [33]. CRP, which is available to clinicians, and procalcitonin, which may be available soon, have been the most studied. A systemic review and meta-analysis of studies that compared procalcitonin and CRP found that, for hospitalized children and adults, procalcitonin was more sensitive (88% versus 67%, respectively) and specific (81% versus 67%%, respectively) in distinguishing bacterial infections from noninfectious causes of inflammation [34]. For distinguishing bacterial from viral infections, procalcitonin was also more sensitive (92% versus 86%, respectively) with similar specificity (73% versus 70%, respectively). However, another such analysis of a larger and more homogenous group of critically ill adults found that procalcitonin could not reliably differentiate sepsis (ie, infection and SIRS) from noninfectious causes of SIRS and had a sensitivity and specificity of only 71% [35]. Procalcitonin may be useful as a prognostic marker. One study found that a high maximum and increase for day 1 of procalcitonin are independent predictors of mortality in mostly adults admitted to the ICU, but initial levels of procalcitonin, and levels or increases in CRP and total peripheral WBC, were not [36].

Establishing a definitive microbial etiology of severe sepsis/septic shock is difficult during ED evaluation. Nonetheless, identification of the organism(s) and antimicrobial susceptibilities can be important in subsequent management. Obtaining appropriate cultures before antimicrobial treatment (ie, when not associated with an unreasonable delay in therapy) optimizes pathogen identification. However, the former approach to withhold empiric therapy because of concern for obscuring a specific etiologic diagnosis has given way to emphasis on broad-spectrum antimicrobial therapy as soon as possible once there is a reasonable suspicion of sepsis/septic shock to optimize patient outcomes.

The recommended practice is to culture at or above 20 mL of blood divided evenly into aerobic and anaerobic bottles [37]. Blood culture yield increases with greater blood volume obtained [38]. The total volume appears to be more important than timing or use of multiple sites [39,40]. However, there is some incremental yield with multiple specimens, and it may also be useful in distinguishing true pathogens from contaminants [41,42]. Therefore, patients being evaluated for severe sepsis/septic shock should have at least a pair (two full volume sets) of blood cultures obtained. For suspected indwelling line infection, the catheter should be removed as soon as possible and the tip cultured.

Selection of other culture sites for specimens should be based on the clinical scenario. The most common sites of infection causing severe sepsis/septic shock are pulmonary, genitourinary, intra-abdominal, skin, and indwelling lines. Urine cultures are easily obtained, and are appropriate in most patients unless there is an obvious alternate source. Culture and gram stain of sputum has low overall yield but is recommended for patients admitted to the ICU with pneumonia [43]. Any purulent material from skin and soft-tissue infections and other normally sterile fluids (eg, joint, cerebrospinal, and pleural fluid) should be obtained for gram stain and culture if there is evidence of localized infection. Urinary testing of pneumococcal and Legionella antigens is recommended now for patients being admitted to the ICU, those who have failed outpatient treatment, and those with comorbidities [43].

Early hemodynamic optimization

In 2001, a trial of early hemodynamic resuscitation to normal physiologic parameters, or early goal-directed therapy (EGDT), was conducted in ED patients with severe sepsis/septic shock and revealed a significant mortality reduction [11]. This clinical trial resulted in recommendations that were central to initiatives to improve outcomes in patients with severe sepsis/septic shock, such as the Surviving Sepsis Campaign [1]. EGDT is an algorithmic approach within the first 6 hours of disease recognition that diverges from standard management primarily by increasing oxygen content (with blood transfusion) and cardiac contractility (with inotropes) to optimize oxygen delivery as measured by oxygen saturation of venous blood from an upper central vein. Specifically, patients are managed by (1) fluid resuscitation with either crystalloid or colloid to achieve a central venous pressure (CVP) goal of 8 to 12 mm Hg; (2) vasoactive agents to achieve a MAP goal of 65 to 90 mm Hg; (3) blood transfusion to a hematocrit at or greater than 30%; (4) inotrope therapy; and (5) intubation, sedation, and paralysis as necessary to achieve a $ScvO_2$ of at or greater than 70% as measured by continuous central venous monitoring (Fig. 1).

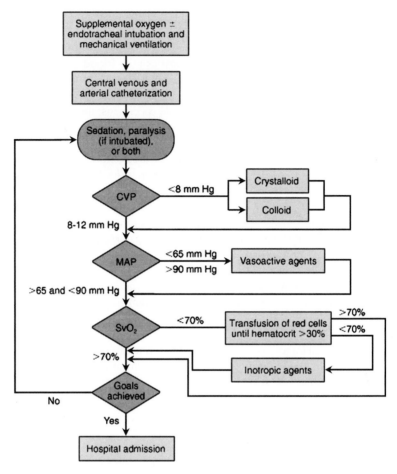

Fig. 1. Early goal-directed therapy protocol. (*From* Rivers E, Nguyen B, Havstad S, et al. Early goal-directed therapy in the treatment of severe sepsis and septic shock. N Engl J Med 2001;345(19):1368–77; with permission.)

In this trial, the efficacy of EGDT was examined in 263 patients with infection associated with hypotension after a fluid bolus and/or serum lactate at or greater than 4 mmol/L and who were randomly assigned to receive standard resuscitation or EGDT (133 control versus 130 EGDT) in the ED before ICU transfer. Largely on the basis of this trial, serum lactate levels are increasingly relied on to screen patients who appear at clinical risk for severe sepsis/septic shock. ICU physicians were blinded to patient study assignment and ED care. During the first 6 hours in the ED, the EGDT group had significantly greater amounts of fluid therapy than the control group (5.0 versus 3.5 L), red blood cell transfusion (64.1 versus 18.5%), and inotrope (ie, dobutamine) administration (13.7 versus 0.8%).

The primary outcome variable, in-hospital mortality, was 46.5% in the control group versus 30.5% in the EGDT group (relative reduction in mortality rate of 34.4%; relative risk [RR] 0.58; 95% CI 0.38–0.87; $P = .009$). Organ dysfunction scores were significantly better in the EGDT group during the first 72 hours; and among patients who survived to hospital discharge, EGDT resulted in a significant 3.8 days shorter hospital length of stay ($P = .04$).

Several limitations of this investigation have been identified, and include the potential for subsequent ICU caregivers to become aware of the patient's prior treatment assignment (such as on account of the unusual and frequent practice of early blood transfusion in the EGDT group). This was a single-site investigation of urban ED patients, and EGDT has not been similarly studied in other centers or settings (eg, for patients in the hospital), although reports of implementation of EGDT and comparison of patient outcomes with those of historical controls support its effectiveness [44–47]. Concerns about the appropriateness and inability to discern the individual effects of specific interventions/strategies that were bundled in EGDT have been raised [48]. As more ED patients are screened with lactate levels, particularly from peripheral venous sites, patients with elevated levels tend to have lower mortality rates than patients with these same levels (ie, ≥ 4 mmol/L) found in selective clinical trials, and thus, the results seen with EGDT may not be seen in other such patients with elevated lactate levels [28]. The validation of this study is planned through a multicenter study called Protocolized Care of Early Septic Shock (PROCESS), which is funded by the National Institutes of Health.

Pending further study, EGDT is recommended. Although this approach has been slow to be incorporated into standard practice [49], establishing protocols and order sets have facilitated its use [5,50,51]. Monitoring of central venous oxygen saturation can be accomplished continuously using a specific catheter or by serial sampling of venous blood gases. In the absence of invasive monitoring, aggressive fluid administration similar to the amounts given in the EGDT study group (which can be guided by bedside ultrasound evaluation of CVP) [52], assessment of serial blood counts and early transfusion, and addition of dobutamine for pressor-unresponsive shock is recommended. In addition to following standard hemodynamic and organ function parameters, serial lactate levels may be useful in determining response to therapy [29].

Antimicrobial therapy

Timeliness and in vitro antimicrobial activity

In light of the dramatic reduction in mortality observed with the advent of modern antimicrobial therapy, it would be unethical to randomize patients with severe sepsis/septic shock either to receive antimicrobials immediately or after some period of delay, or to antimicrobials expected to have or not have in vitro activity against anticipated pathogens.

Several retrospective cohort studies of bacteremic patients with community-acquired infections have examined the institution of "appropriate" empirical antimicrobials with respect to mortality (ie, those given with in vitro activity against the blood culture isolate within 24 to 48 h of specimen collection versus inappropriate antimicrobials) [53–71]. These studies had variable proportions of patients with community-acquired infections and shock. Most studies found a lower mortality associated with the institution of appropriate antimicrobials and support the importance of accurately predicting the bacterial etiology of sepsis and the associated antimicrobial susceptibility when choosing empirical antimicrobials.

The causation associated with an alleged "delay" to administer antibiotics in relation to outcome is a frequent and contentious medical–legal issue in serious infectious diseases cases. Although studies have looked at antimicrobial administration within 24 to 48 hours of blood culture collection, there are only limited data on the effect of shorter antibiotic delays for various types of serious infections within the typical timeframe of ED care (ie, several hours). Among patients with meningococcemia, Cartwright and colleagues [72] found lower mortality associated with antibiotic administration by general practitioners before transfer to the hospital compared with administration at the hospital, but these differences were not statistically significant.

Among hospitalized patients, Kumar and colleagues [73] found that survival was inversely proportional to time to initiation of antibiotics from the onset of septic shock, with an approximately linear 8%/h absolute decline. This relationship was reported in an investigation of ED patients hospitalized with various severities of sepsis, and delay in initiation of adequate antibiotic therapy was also directly related to an increase in the Sequential Organ Failure Assessment (SOFA) score. However, this relationship was poorly predictive of complications in individual patients [70]. A murine model of *Escherichia coli*-induced septic shock found that the duration of hypotension before antibiotic initiation was a critical determinant of survival, with an inflection point at about 12 to 15 hours when serum lactate levels began to rise. At or before 12 hours, mortality was less than 20%, but at or after 15 hours mortality was greater than 85% [74]. Therefore, it would appear that earlier antibiotics could have a marked effect on improved survival if administered before the onset of severe sepsis/septic shock as evidenced by the appearance of lactic acidosis. However, once this condition is established, mortality rates are substantially higher and the relationship between time to initiation of antibiotics and survival is incremental and much less marked. Therefore, in any one patient with severe sepsis/septic shock, the effect of a few hours of delay on mortality or sepsis-related complications is small and difficult to predict.

The Surviving Sepsis Campaign, an initiative of the European Society of Intensive Care Medicine, the International Sepsis Forum, and the Society of

Critical Care Medicine, recommended "Intravenous antibiotic therapy should be started within the *first hour* of *recognition* of severe sepsis" [1]. In practice, recognition of severe sepsis/septic shock and other infectious disease emergencies and the provision of antibiotics appear to take several hours. For example, studies of suspected bacterial meningitis have found that median times from ED registration to initiation of antibiotics were 3 to 4 hours [75,76], and another study found the median time from the onset of septic shock in hospitalized patients to antibiotic initiation was 6 hours [73]. A recent ED-based guideline concluded that

> Although there are insufficient data to conclude that delays on the order of hours are deleterious, administration of antibiotics within the timeframe of ED care and as soon as possible once there is a reasonable suspicion of severe sepsis/septic shock will likely increase the chance of favorable outcome compared with later administration [5].

This recommendation is similar to that of the Infectious Diseases Association of America (IDSA) for initiation of antibiotics for ED patients with community-acquired pneumonia being admitted to the hospital [43].

Infection site and bacterial etiology

As culture results are not available within the timeframe of ED care, anticipated pathogens must be predicted based on the infection site and past studies of the associated etiologies. Most studies describing the bacteriology and sites of infection in severe sepsis/septic shock include a combination of community- and hospital-acquired infections [77–93]. The common sites of infection are lung (35%), abdomen (21%), urinary tract (13%), skin and soft tissue (7%), other site (8%), and unknown primary site (16%) (compiled from 16 studies between 1963 and 1998 that included 8667 patients). Among patients older than 65 years of age, a urinary tract source is the most common infection site [62,94].

Although several studies describe community-acquired bacteremia, in most investigations only a fraction of patients had severe sepsis/septic shock. In one multicenter study of 339 patients admitted to the ICU with community-acquired bacteremia, with sepsis in 86 cases (25%), severe sepsis in 69 cases (20%), and septic shock in 184 cases (55%), the sites of infection were lung (21%), abdomen (20%), urinary tract (20%), endocarditis (4%), other (10%), and bloodstream infection without known primary source (25%) [71]. The most common pathogens were *Escherichia coli* (25%), *Streptococcus pneumoniae* (16%), and *Staphylococcus aureus* (14%); about 4% were due to potentially multidrug-resistant, gram-negative bacilli such as *Pseudomonas aeruginosa* and *Acinetobacter baumannii*. In another study, conducted in 1997–2000, of 169 bacteremic patients admitted from nursing homes (only 20% had hypotension), the most common pathogens were *E coli* (27%), *S aureus* (18%, about one-third methicillin-resistant *S aureus* [MRSA]), and *Proteus* spp (13%); about 3% of episodes were caused by

P aeruginosa [94]. In general, multidrug-resistant, gram-negative bacteria such as *P aeruginosa* are rare causes of community-acquired bacteremia and severe/sepsis and septic shock. However, as more community patients with health care exposures present to the ED, these multidrug-resistant infections may become more common. Of note, for *Psuedomonal* bacteremia, the association of appropriate antibiotics and improved survival has not been clearly established, perhaps owing to overwhelming importance of host factors [95].

Antimicrobial susceptibility

Because of the association of survival with an initial antimicrobial regimen that possesses in vitro activity against the offending bacterial pathogen, it is important to understand current antimicrobial resistance patterns and trends that may help anticipate future resistance. To the best of the present authors' knowledge, no series exist for bacterial pathogens and their associated antimicrobial susceptibility patterns among ED patients with severe sepsis/septic shock. However, general antimicrobial susceptibility surveys of the three major pathogens—*E coli*, *S aureus*, and *S pneumoniae*—have been conducted, and some report on community-acquired strains. These studies are often limited by lack of specific knowledge regarding outpatient setting/exposure, prior antimicrobial use, and site of infection. Populations are limited to patients with cultures, and their results describe susceptibility patterns of several years before the time of publication. It is important to understand antimicrobial resistance rates locally; national and international resistance trends may also be helpful. Antimicrobial use by patients within the previous several months is a recognized risk factor for being colonized or infected with a strain resistant to a previously administered antimicrobial and other antimicrobials [96]. Also, it can no longer be assumed that all patients coming through the ED have community-acquired infections, as many come from nursing homes or have recently been exposed to a health care setting and are a risk for unusual multidrug-resistant pathogens.

Although more than 90% of *E coli* isolates (and other *Enterobacteriaceae*) collected in 2000–2001 from hospitalized patients, but not including nursing home residents, in the United States were susceptible to aminoglycosides, fluoroquinolones, and advanced-generation cephalosporins [97], no one class of gram-negative antimicrobials was universally active, with higher resistance rates for *P aeruginosa*, *Acinetobacter baumannii*, or extended beta-lactamase–producing species. For example, for *P aeruginosa,* susceptibility rates were gentamicin, 79%; ciprofloxacin, 73%; ceftazidime, 81%; imipenem, 84%; and piperacillin-tazobactam, 90%. Another report of clinical *P aeruginosa* isolates found that ciprofloxacin and levofloxacin provided very similar improvements in susceptibility when combined with anti-pseudomonal beta-lactam as compared with adding gentamicin, increasing the percentage of susceptible isolates by an absolute amount of 3% to 8% [98].

The prevalence of community-acquired strains of *S pneumoniae* with penicillin, macrolide, and/or trimethoprim-sulfamethoxazole resistance has significantly increased in the last decade. Resistance rates to third-generation cephalosporins such as ceftriaxone and cefotaxime are still low, ranging from 3% to 5%, especially since the cutoff above which a minimal inhibitory concentration would be defined as "resistant" was revised upward (ie, from ≥ 2 μg/mL to ≥ 4 μg/mL) [99,100]. Resistance rates to respiratory fluoroquinolones are similarly low but are increasing in North America [101]. There are no reports of *S pneumoniae* with in vitro resistance to vancomycin or newer gram-positive active agents.

Community-associated methicillin-resistant *S aureus* (CA-MRSA) infections are rapidly increasing and appear now to be the most common pathogen isolated in community-acquired skin and soft-tissue infections [102]. CA-MRSA has also been associated with severe sepsis and pneumonia, primarily in pediatric patients [103]. Antimicrobials with consistent in vitro activity against CA-MRSA isolates include vancomycin, trimethoprim-sulfamethoxazole, daptomycin, tigecycline, and linezolid. Most isolates are resistant to macrolides and quinolones, and some are resistant to tetracycline, including doxycycline. In general, clindamycin has good in vitro activity against CA-MRSA [102,104]; however, some centers report high rates of clindamycin resistance [105,106], which has also been seen in some risk groups—specifically, men who have sex with men. Inducible clindamycin resistance exists among some CA-MRSA strains and has been associated with clinical failures [107]. Health care-associated strains of MRSA are still a common cause of infections in patients who have certain high risk exposures; for example, among dialysis patients with invasive infections in 2005, 80% of MRSA strains were of health care origin [108]. A recent concern is increasing vancomycin minimum inhibitory concentrations to methicillin-susceptible *S. aureus* (MSSA) and MRSA and its association with decreased clinical efficacy [109–111]. Also, certain gram-positive active antibiotics—specifically, clindamycin and linezolid—appear to inhibit the expression of virulence-associated exotoxin genes, thereby suppressing toxin production, and also have the capacity for bacterial killing of stationary-phase growth organisms that cell-wall active agents lack [112]. Antibiotics with these properties may be preferred to treat infections caused by toxin-producing gram-positive pathogens.

Empirical antimicrobial consideration and recommendations

Antimicrobial recommendations for patients with severe sepsis/septic shock are based on pathogen prevalence and susceptibility patterns from community-acquired infections, as comparative studies among severe sepsis/septic shock patients do not exist. The recommendations are also based on the principle that, because this subgroup of patients has a predicted mortality of 20% to 50%, and in vitro activity of the treatment regimen against the causative bacteria is generally associated with lower mortality, the empirical regimens should be sufficiently broad so that there is little chance that the offending pathogen will not be effectively covered. Compared with the potential benefit of this approach, promotion of antimicrobial resistance is a minor risk, and the antimicrobial regimens can be tailored back once pathogen identification and susceptibilities are available in a few days. If the site of a community-acquired infection has not been identified, initial empirical therapy should target E coli, S aureus (including MRSA), and S pneumoniae, and to the extent the site of infection is identified, empirical regimens should be more specific.

For E coli and other gram-negative bacteria, two potentially active antibiotics from different classes are recommended as no one class of agents has universal activity, particularly considering the growing number of community-residing patients with health care exposures. In this case, two agents are advised to ensure that at least one has in vitro activity, as the use of dually active or synergistic combinations has not been clearly associated with improved outcomes [113]. Fortunately, for patients presenting from the community, potentially multidrug-resistant gram-negative infections, such as due to P aeruginosa, are rare. Ceftriaxone, which is consistently stocked in EDs, is active against approximately 98% of E coli bloodstream isolates in North America, and provides adequate gram-negative coverage of most presentations associated with non-health care settings [97]. There appears to be comparable enhancement of anti-pseudomonal beta-lactam activity with levofloxacin and ciprofloxacin, as with gentamicin, providing another option to avoid potential aminoglycoside-associated nephrotoxicity and ototoxicity. Levofloxacin could thus be used as part of a general regimen for coverage of pneumonia and as an additional gram-negative active drug.

For intra-abdominal and complicated urinary tract infection etiologies, enterococci must be considered potential pathogens in the setting of severe sepsis/ septic shock, and the addition of an aminoglycoside to a beta-lactam or vancomycin (or another broadly active gram-positive agent) should be strongly considered, as the combination has been associated with more reliable cure with enterococcal endocarditis than beta-lactam monotherapy [114]. Anaerobic coverage is additionally recommended for abdominal/pelvic infections.

For presumed staphylococcal infections, vancomycin has traditionally been recommended; however, there are increasing concerns because of rising vancomycin minimal inhibitory concentrations associated with higher rates of clinical failure and evidence of inferior efficacy compared with beta-lactams for treatment of MSSA infections [109,111]. Based on these concerns, the addition of a semisynthetic penicillin, such as nafallin to vancomycin, should strongly be considered when a staphylococcal etiology is suspected [115]. Linezolid has been associated with higher clinical cure rates compared with vancomycin for complicated MRSA skin and soft-tissue infections and nosocomial and ventilator-associated pneumonia on subset analyses. Linezolid also has been used effectively to treat serious infections for which vancomycin failed; however, it has not been sufficiently evaluated for blood-stream infections [116–118]. Clindamycin or linezolid is recommended to be included in empirical regimes to treat severe skin and soft-tissue infections such as necrotizing fasciitis to enhance killing of organisms with stationary growth and to decrease toxin production.

All of the recommended regimens for staphylococcal infection would provide coverage for infection due to *S pneumoniae,* including infections due to strains resistant to beta-lactams and fluoroquinolones. For suspected severe pneumonia, a respiratory quinolone, such as levofloxacin or moxifloxacin, which would also provide atypical coverage, along with an anti-staphylococcal agent, is recommended [43]. For presumed bacterial meningitis, ceftriaxone (or cefotaxime) and vancomycin are recommended.

Specific empiric drug regimens are listed as examples to facilitate implementation and, in part, were chosen based on current availability in EDs. The inclusion of specific drugs is not meant to imply that these are the exclusive drugs of choice. Reasonable alternative therapies are footnoted (Table 1).

Source control

Early detection of the site of infection determines the presumptive microbiologic etiology, guiding selection of empirical therapy as described above, and identifies the need for critical source control measures. Thus, the emergency physician has a challenging task to orchestrate initial respiratory and hemodynamic resuscitation, expedite antibiotic administration, simultaneously hunt for a source of infection, and involve appropriate consultants. While the patient is being stabilized, in addition to laboratory investigations, portable plain X rays and bedside ultrasonography, which is being used more routinely by emergency physicians, can help to quickly identify pneumonia/empyema, soft-tissue gas, ascites, cholecystitis, visceral abscess, and urinary tract obstruction associated with urosepsis. When the patient is stabilized, further investigation with rapid spiral CT scanning (eg, abdomen/pelvis) can be done if necessary. Source control measures include abscess and empyema drainage, tissue débridement (eg, for necrotizing fasciitis), removal of infected prostheses (eg, for intravenous lines), dilatation and curettage (eg, for septic abortion), and bypass of obstructions (eg, for urinary tract lesions). Many of these interventions can be done relatively noninvasively, such as with percutaneous drainage of intra-abdominal abscesses. Early source control has been associated with decreased morbidity and mortality, and thus, investigations and interventions, when these can be done with reasonably safety, should be pursued urgently after resuscitation is instituted [119,120].

Recombinant human-activated protein C

Cleavage of protein C by thrombin associated with thrombomodulin generates activated protein C, which has potent anticoagulant,

Table 1
Examples of empirical antimicrobials recommended for adult emergency department patients with severe sepsis and septic shock

Sepsis source	Recommended antimicrobial regimen (standard adult dosing)	Comments
Unknown source	Vancomycin[a] 1 g q 12 h, levofloxacin[b] 750 mg q 24 h, and ceftriaxone[b] 2 g q 24 h	Search for a source of infection with physical examination, chest radiograph, bedside ultrasound, and urinalysis; consider abdominal/pelvic CT if no source found
Community-acquired pneumonia	Vancomycin[a] 1 g q 12 h, levofloxacin[c] 750 mg q 24 h, and ceftriaxone 2 g q 24 h	Evaluate pleural fluid and drain empyema if present. Obtain echocardiogram if endocarditis with septic emboli are suspected (eg, in intravenous drug users).
Meningitis	Vancomycin 1 g q 12 h and ceftriaxone 2 g q 12 h (and ampicillin 2 g q 4 h if immunocompromised or >50 years of age) after dexamethasone 10 mg IV q 6 h	Administer acyclovir (10 mg/kg q 8 h) if herpes encephalitis suspected (eg, altered mental status or focal neurological abnormalities)
Urinary tract infection	Piperacillin/tazobactam 4.5 g q 8 h and gentamicin 7 mg/kg q 24 h (see Comments for treatment options)	Complicated urinary tract infections may be caused by Enterococcus species, Pseudomonas aeruginosa, or Staphylococcus aureus (non-nitrite producers) for which piperacillin/tazobactam and aminoglycoside are preferred. If urine nitrite production or gram stain suggest Enterobacteriaceae, fluoroquinolones or advanced-generation cephalosporins can be substituted for gentamicin. Obtain imaging to rule out obstruction as soon as possible.

| Intra-abdominal/pelvic infection | Piperacillin/tazobactam[d] 4.5 g q 8 h and gentamicin[b] 7 mg/kg q 24 h | Obtain surgical consultation for surgical exploration, or, if indicated, imaging to identify infection focus and potential for percutaneous or open drainage |
| Skin and soft- tissue infection/necrotizing infection | Vancomycin[e] 1 g q 12 h, piperacillin/tazobactam[d] 4.5 g q 8 h, and clindamycin[e] 900 mg q 8 h | For suspected necrotizing infections, obtain surgical consultation for tissue debridement as soon as possible |

Dosages are for ~70-kg adults with normal renal and hepatic function.

[a] Strongly consider adding an antistaphylococcal semisynthetic penicillin, such as nafcillin; may substitute daptomycin (not for pneumonia).

[b] May substitute gram-negative agents (from different classes), including piperacillin/tazobactam, ceftazidime, cefepime, aztreonam, imipenem, meropenem, ciprofloxacin, or an aminoglycoside. For patients with health care exposure and/or immunocompromise, an antipseudomonal gram-negative agent should be substituted for ceftriaxone.

[c] May substitute moxifloxacin.

[d] May substitute imipenem or meropenem.

[e] May substitute linezolid for vancomycin and clindamycin.

profibrinolytic, anti-inflammatory, and anti-apoptotic effects. Activated protein C cleavage is down-regulated in sepsis. PROWESS, a multicenter, international, placebo-controlled study, investigated the ability of drotrecogin alfa (activated) to reduce 28-day mortality [22]. Study entry required clinical evidence of infection, presence of a systemic inflammatory response syndrome, and at least one sepsis-induced organ dysfunction present for less than 48 hours. Organ dysfunction included fluid-unresponsive hypotension (systolic blood pressure ≤ 90 mm Hg or MAP ≤ 70 mm Hg ≥ 1 h), decreased urine output, hypoxemia, lactic acidosis, or thrombocytopenia. A total of 1690 patients were enrolled, and 28-day mortality rates were reduced from 30.8% in the placebo group to 24.7% in the treatment group (relative reduction in mortality rate of 19.8%; RR 0.80; 95% CI 0.69–0.94; $P = .005$). Benefit from drotrecogin alfa (activated) was present in patients with various etiologies of bacterial infection and in those in whom culture results were negative.

Survival benefit with drotrecogin alfa (activated) was associated with higher severity of illness, described by either the number of sepsis-induced organ failures or the Acute Physiology and Chronic Health Evaluation II (APACHE II) score, which incorporates laboratory, clinical, age, and chronic illness components [121]. In analyses prespecified in the protocol, drotrecogin alfa (activated) was found to reduce absolute mortality by 13% in septic patients with APACHE II scores of 25 or greater (or ≥ 2 sepsis-induced organ dysfunctions), and the drug was approved by the US Food and Drug Administration for use only for patients meeting this criterion [122]. Recent data from the Administration of Drotrecogin Alfa (Activated) in Early Stage Severe Sepsis (ADDRESS) trial in patients with single-organ dysfunction or an APACHE II score below 25 showed that these patients did not benefit from drotrecogin alfa (activated) [123]. In the same study, patients with recent surgery within 30 days and single-organ dysfunction who received drotrecogin alfa (activated) had higher 28-day mortality compared with patients receiving placebo. Multiple patient populations, such as those with end-stage liver disease or requiring hemodialysis for end-stage renal disease (in which severe sepsis/septic shock is common), were excluded from the PROWESS study. The efficacy of drotrecogin alfa (activated) in such groups is currently unknown. Most important, patients with high risk for bleeding were excluded owing to concerns surrounding the anticoagulant properties of drotrecogin alfa (activated). A recently published randomized, double-blind, placebo-controlled trial examining the efficacy of drotrecogin alfa (activated) in pediatric patients was discontinued because there was no improvement compared with placebo in mortality or resolution of organ dysfunction over 14 days [124].

As expected, given the anticoagulant properties of drotrecogin alfa (activated), the major clinical risk with its use is bleeding. Severe bleeding episodes considered to be life-threatening or requiring the transfusion of more than three units of packed red blood cells per day for 2 consecutive days were present in 3.5% of patients receiving drotrecogin alfa (activated) in the PROWESS study, as compared with 2.0% in the placebo group ($P = .06$) [22]. Intracranial hemorrhage occurred during the infusion period in 0.2% of the drotrecogin alfa (activated)-treated group in the PROWESS study, and has been reported to occur in 0.5% of patients during drotrecogin alfa (activated) infusion in subsequent controlled and open-label trials [125]. If all bleeding events are considered, administration of drotrecogin alfa (activated) approximately doubles the risk [122]. Additional analyses have also demonstrated that platelet counts below 30,000/mm^3 are associated with higher frequency of severe bleeding with drotrecogin alfa (activated) [125]. The timing of drotrecogin alfa (activated) administration may be also affect outcomes. In the PROWESS study, the time from organ dysfunction to start of drug infusion was 17.5 ± 12.8 hours [22]. In a global open-label, single-arm study (Extended Evaluation of Recombinant Human Activated Protein C—ENHANCE) that enrolled 2378 patients, those who received drotrecogin alfa (activated) within 24 hours of recognition of organ dysfunction had a 28-day mortality rate of 22.9% compared with 27.4% in those who received it after 24 hours ($P = .01$) [126]. Evaluation of five clinical trials from 4459 patients also suggested that earlier treatment was associated with a modest benefit [127]. The absolute contraindications to administration of drotrecogin alfa (activated) are the following:

Active internal bleeding
Recent hemorrhagic stroke within 3 months
Recent intracranial or intraspinal surgery, or severe head trauma within 2 months
Trauma with an increased risk of life-threatening bleeding
Presence of an epidural catheter
Intracranial neoplasm, mass lesion, or evidence of cerebral herniation
Known hypersensitivity to drotrecogin alfa (activated)

A concern regarding the efficacy of drotrecogin alfa (activated) is that the protocol used in PROWESS was modified approximately halfway through the study [128]. After entry criteria were revised to exclude certain high-risk patients, and a new placebo composition and a new cell bank to produce drotrecogin alfa (activated) were introduced, there was improved benefit shown in the treatment group. The trial may have been difficult to blind as the treatment was associated with excessive bleeding, including with venipunctures. A recent retrospective subset analysis of PROWESS study patients with community-acquired pneumonia found that the 90-day survival benefit was largely due to an 18.1% absolute reduction in mortality in patients with inadequate antibiotic therapy (65.2% to 47.1%), being limited to only 4% in patients with adequate antimicrobial treatment (37% to 33%), further highlighting the importance of appropriate empirical antibiotics [129]. Also, use evaluations of drotrecogin alfa (activated) have found adverse effect and mortality rates higher than in the original

PROWESS study [130]. A new phase III placebo-controlled trial of drotre-cogin alfa (activated) has been announced that will be conducted in patients within the currently indicated population (adults with severe sepsis at high risk of death) and will use the current standard of care for severe sepsis [131].

At present, in patients with severe sepsis/septic shock, drotrecogin alfa (activated) should be considered when the APACHE II score is 25 or greater for those who have received appropriate antimicrobial therapy and have not responded to initial hemodynamic optimization, such as by early–goal-directed therapy.

Supplemental steroids

The physiologic response to sepsis is increased levels of stress hormones such as cortisol. Some patients with septic shock will have inadequate ad-renal reserve manifested by an inadequate response when challenged with adrenocorticotropic hormone (ACTH) or corticotrophin-releasing hor-mone. Relative adrenal insufficiency, defined as an increase in serum corti-sol of less than or equal to 9 µg/dL 1 hour after administration of 250 µg of ACTH, is present in the majority of mechanically ventilated patients who have fluid-refractory septic shock [132]. The presence of inadequate adrenal reserve, as determined by response to ACTH, is associated with worse outcomes, including higher mortality rates and prolonged require-ments for vasopressors as compared with an adequate cortisol response to ACTH [133].

Although previous investigations did not demonstrate a beneficial effect of large doses of synthetic corticosteroids for patients with septic shock [134–136], a multicenter, placebo-controlled study found lower supplemen-tal stress doses of natural corticosteroids to be associated with improved outcomes. Annane and colleagues [137] studied severely ill patients as de-fined by more than 1 hour of fluid unresponsive hypotension and an above 5-µg/kg/min requirement for dopamine or other vasopressors, such as nor-epinephrine or epinephrine. Additional entry criteria included a requirement for mechanical ventilation and evidence of at least one additional sepsis-induced organ dysfunction such as urine output of less than 0.5 mL/kg/h, serum lactate greater than 2 mmol/L, or hypoxemia ($PaO_2/FiO_2 < 280$). Following an ACTH stimulation test at study entry, subjects were random-ized to placebo or corticosteroids (hydrocortisone 50 mg intravenous every 6 hours and the mineralocorticoid, 9α-fludrocortisone 50 µg, once daily by mouth) for 7 days. Administration of corticosteroids resulted in a 28-day mortality of 63% in the placebo group compared with 53% in the treatment group who did not respond appropriately to ACTH (relative reduction in mortality rate of 16%; RR, 0.83; 95% CI, 0.66–1.04; $P = .04$). Time on vasopressors was also significantly improved when low-dose corticosteroids were administered to septic shock patients with inadequate adrenal reserve.

Corticosteroid administration was not associated with increases in infectious complications, gastrointestinal bleeding, or mental status changes. Of note, there was a nonstatistically significant increased mortality rate among corticosteroid-treated patients compared with placebo treated with an appropriate cortisol response to ACTH (61% versus 53%, respectively). This potential detrimental effect is concerning when considering this treatment for ED patients, who are generally at an earlier stage of illness and may be more likely to have adrenal responsiveness.

A recently completed multicenter trial, Corticosteroid Therapy in Septic Shock, by the European Society of Intensive Care Medicine, did not validate the efficacy of low-dose corticosteroid supplementation [138]. Among 499 patients randomized to hydrocortisone 50 mg every 6 hours for 5 days, then 50 mg every 12 hours for 3 days, followed by 50 mg every 24 hours for 2 days (no fludrocortisone was given) or placebo, there was no significant difference in mortality rate (34% versus 31%, respectively), which did not vary by responder status. Although entry criteria were similar, the study differed from that of Annane and colleagues [137] in that the overall mortality was lower (38% versus 59%, respectively) and fewer patients had adrenal unresponsiveness (47% versus 77%, respectively). In addition, there was a nonstatistically significant trend toward higher rates of superinfection in the corticosteroid arm (33% versus 26%, respectively). In light of these findings, and the greater likelihood of adrenal responsiveness in ED patients with severe sepsis/septic shock, supplemental steroids are not recommended unless frank adrenal insufficiency is suspected.

Other therapeutic considerations

Low-tidal volume mechanical ventilation

A large, multicenter trial of patients with acute respiratory distress syndrome, the majority of whom had sepsis or pneumonia as the associated etiology, showed that the use of low-tidal volume mechanical ventilation reduced mortality rates from 39.8% in the conventionally ventilated patients to 31% in those who received low-tidal volume ventilation (relative reduction in mortality rate of 22.1%; 95% CI % for the absolute difference between groups, 2.4–15.3) [139]. In this study, patients with acute lung injury were randomized to either low (6 mL/kg based on ideal body weight) or conventional (12 mL/kg based on ideal body weight) tidal volumes. In the low-tidal volume group, airway plateau pressures were kept at or below 30 cm H_2O by decreasing the tidal volume to as low as 4 mL/kg if necessary, and in the conventional-tidal volume group, airway plateau pressures were not allowed to be above 50 cm H_2O. Therefore, for although this was not a study of severe sepsis/septic shock requiring mechanical ventilation, a low-tidal volume/low-pressure strategy is recommended.

Tight glucose control

A prospective, randomized, controlled trial of adults admitted to a surgical ICU and receiving mechanical ventilation compared intensive insulin therapy to maintain a blood glucose of 80 to 110 mg/dL with an insulin-only regimen if the blood glucose exceeded 215 mg/dL and maintenance between 180 and 200 mg/dL. A beneficial effect was associated with tight glucose control compared with conventional treatment in terms of mortality rate in the ICU (4.6% versus 8.0%, respectively, relative reduction in mortality rate of 42%, 95% CI, 22 to 62%, $P < .04$), particularly due to multiple organ failure with proven sepsis (1.0% versus 4.2%, respectively) [140]. However, more recently a similar trial was conducted among a mixed population of medical ICU patients. No mortality difference was found between patients receiving intensive compared with conventional insulin therapy either in the ICU (24.2% versus 26.8%, respectively, $P = .31$) or in-hospital (37.3% versus 40.0%, respectively, $P = .33$). Intensive insulin therapy was associated with mortality reduction among patients staying at least 3 days in the ICU, because this treatment also was associated with prevention of newly acquired kidney injury, accelerated weaning from mechanical ventilation, and faster ICU and hospital discharge [141]. At present, the use of intensive insulin therapy remains controversial, and as studies of tight glucose control have not been specifically conducted among patients with severe sepsis/septic shock—including in the ED—the efficacy of this approach for this condition is unclear.

Bicarbonate replacement

Patients with severe sepsis/septic shock may have profound metabolic and lactic acidosis. Although bicarbonate replacement can temporarily change the acid-base status toward normal values, controlled trials have found that bicarbonate does not improve hemodynamic parameters; therefore, it is not recommended [142,143].

Summary

With the discovery of new strategies and therapies to optimize the outcome of patients with severe sepsis/septic shock, increasing emphasis is being placed on rapid diagnosis and treatment initiated in the ED. Fig. 2 is an algorithm that summarizes management guidelines for ED care of patients with septic shock/severe sepsis. The goal of diagnosis in the ED is to identify patients with severe sepsis/septic shock (ie, with evidence of organ dysfunctions, lactic acidosis, and fluid nonresponsive hypotension). SIRS criteria and routine tests, such as the peripheral WBC count and differential, are too nonspecific to be useful in this population. The role of new sepsis biomarkers, such as procalcitonin, is currently being evaluated.

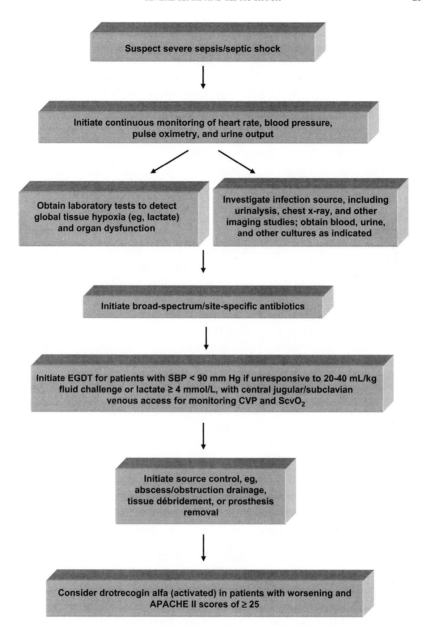

Fig. 2. Summary algorithm of management guidelines for ED care of patients with septic shock/severe sepsis. ACTH, adrenocorticotropic hormone; APACHE, Acute Physiology and Chronic Health Evaluation; CVP, central venous pressure; EGDT, early goal-directed therapy; SBP, systolic blood pressure; ScvO$_2$, central venous oxygen saturation.

EGDT is a hemodynamic resuscitation strategy using fluids, pressors, blood transfusion, inotropes, and mechanical ventilation protocols, as needed, to optimize oxygen delivery. On the basis of one single-center randomized trial, it appears to markedly reduce mortality, and protocols are being promoted in EDs and on hospital and ICU wards while a multicenter validation trial is ongoing.

Empirical antibiotic therapy must now cover MRSA and MSSA, while vancomycin's effectiveness is debated and other gram-positive active agents become available. The addition of nafcillin to vancomycin for empirical staphylococcal coverage is recommended now. Also, no one class of gram-negative active antibiotics is universally active against community-acquired gram-negative pathogens, and thus, two drugs from different classes are recommended. Antibiotic therapy should be initiated as soon as possible once there is a reasonable suspicion of severe sepsis/septic shock. However, it should be recognized that clinical evaluation is dynamic, and along with various processes of care, requires time to establish a reasonably accurate presumptive diagnosis. Once severe sepsis/septic shock is established, the hourly incremental effect of antibiotic delay is small.

Diagnostic testing to identify a source of infection has advanced with the use of bedside ultrasonography in the ED and access to rapid spiral CT, which allows more specific empirical antimicrobial therapy and early surgical source control measures. Patients refractory to these initial interventions may be candidates for recombinant drotrecogin alfa (activated), while concerns persist as to its effectiveness and safety and a new phase III placebo-controlled trial is planned. The initial enthusiasm for supplemental low-dose steroids, based on one positive, single-center randomized trial in mechanically ventilated septic shock patients, has diminished with the recent report of a negative validation trial.

References

[1] Dellinger RP, Carlet JM, Masur H, et al. Surviving sepsis campaign guidelines for management of severe sepsis and septic shock. Crit Care Med 2004;32(3):858–72.
[2] McCaig LF, Burt CW. National Hospital Ambulatory Medical Care Survey: 2001 emergency department summary. Adv Data 2003;335:1–29.
[3] Angus DC, Linde-Zwirble WT, Lidicker J, et al. Epidemiology of severe sepsis in the United States: analysis of incidence, outcome, and associated costs of care. Crit Care Med 2001; 29(7):1303–10.
[4] Wang HE, Shapiro NI, Angus DC, et al. National estimates of severe sepsis in United States emergency departments. Crit Care Med 2007;35(8):1928–36.
[5] Nguyen HB, Rivers EP, Abrahamian FM, et al. Consensus guidelines for the treatment of severe sepsis and septic shock in the emergency department. Ann Emerg Med 2006;48(1):28–54.
[6] American College of Chest Physicians/Society of Critical Care Medicine Consensus Conference. Definitions for sepsis and organ failure and guidelines for the use of innovative therapies in sepsis. Crit Care Med 1992;20(6):864–74.
[7] Levy MM, Fink MP, Marshall JC, et al. 2001 SCCM/ESICM/ACCP/ATS/SIS International Sepsis Definitions Conference. Intensive Care Med 2003;29(4):530–8.

[8] Talan DA. Dear SIRS: it's time to return to sepsis as we have known it [editorial]. Ann Emerg Med 2006;48(5):591–2.

[9] Shapiro NI, Howell MD, Bates DW, et al. The association of sepsis syndrome and organ dysfunction with mortality in emergency department patients with suspected infection. Ann Emerg Med 2006;48(5):583–90.

[10] Dremsizov T, Clermont G, Kellum JA, et al. Severe sepsis in community-acquired pneumonia: when does it happen, and do systemic inflammatory response syndrome criteria help predict course? Chest 2006;129(4):968–78.

[11] Rivers E, Nguyen B, Havstad S, et al. Early goal-directed therapy in the treatment of severe sepsis and septic shock. N Engl J Med 2001;345(19):1368–77.

[12] Rangel-Frausto MS, Pittet D, Costigan M, et al. The natural history of the systemic inflammatory response syndrome (SIRS). A prospective study. JAMA 1995;273(2):117–23.

[13] Cornbleet PJ. Clinical utility of the band count. Clin Lab Med 2002;22(1):101–36.

[14] Novak RW. The beleaguered band count. Clin Lab Med 1993;13(4):895–903.

[15] Wenz B, Gennis P, Canova C, et al. The clinical utility of the leukocyte differential in emergency medicine. Am J Clin Pathol 1986;86(3):298–303.

[16] Ardron MJ, Westengard JC, Dutcher TF. Band neutrophil counts are unnecessary for the diagnosis of infection in patients with normal total leukocyte counts. Am J Clin Pathol 1994;102(5):646–9.

[17] Callaham M. Inaccuracy and expense of the leukocyte count in making urgent clinical decisions. Ann Emerg Med 1986;15(7):774–81.

[18] Kuppermann N, Walton EA. Immature neutrophils in the blood smears of young febrile children. Arch Pediatr Adolesc Med 1999;153(3):261–6.

[19] Shapiro NI, Wolfe RE, Moore RB, et al. Mortality in Emergency Department Sepsis (MEDS) score: a prospectively derived and validated clinical prediction rule. Crit Care Med 2003;31(3):670–5.

[20] Fine MJ, Auble TE, Yealy DM, et al. A prediction rule to identify low-risk patients with community-acquired pneumonia. N Engl J Med 1997;336(4):243–50.

[21] Vanderschueren S, De Weerdt A, Malbrain M, et al. Thrombocytopenia and prognosis in intensive care. Crit Care Med 2000;28(6):1871–6.

[22] Bernard GR, Vincent JL, Laterre PF, et al. Efficacy and safety of recombinant human activated protein C for severe sepsis. N Engl J Med 2001;344(10):699–709.

[23] Kinasewitz GT, Yan SB, Basson B, et al. Universal changes in biomarkers of coagulation and inflammation occur in patients with severe sepsis, regardless of causative micro-organism [ISRCTN74215569]. Crit Care 2004;8(2):R82–90.

[24] Levraut J, Bounatirou T, Ichai C, et al. Reliability of anion gap as an indicator of blood lactate in critically ill patients. Intensive Care Med 1997;23(4):417–22.

[25] Iberti TJ, Leibowitz AB, Papadakos PJ, et al. Low sensitivity of the anion gap as a screen to detect hyperlactatemia in critically ill patients. Crit Care Med 1990;18(3):275–7.

[26] Abramson D, Scalea TM, Hitchcock R, et al. Lactate clearance and survival following injury. J Trauma 1993;35(4):584–8 [discussion 588–9].

[27] Bakker J, Gris P, Coffernils M, et al. Serial blood lactate levels can predict the development of multiple organ failure following septic shock. Am J Surg 1996;171(2):221–6.

[28] Shapiro NI, Howell MD, Talmor D, et al. Serum lactate as a predictor of mortality in emergency department patients with infection. Ann Emerg Med 2005;45(5):524–8.

[29] Nguyen HB, Rivers EP, Knoblich BP, et al. Early lactate clearance is associated with improved outcome in severe sepsis and septic shock. Crit Care Med 2004;32(8):1637–42.

[30] Weil MH, Michaels S, Rackow EC. Comparison of blood lactate concentrations in central venous, pulmonary artery, and arterial blood. Crit Care Med 1987;15(5):489–90.

[31] Murdoch IA, Turner C, Dalton RN. Arterial or mixed venous lactate measurement in critically ill children. Is there a difference? Acta Paediatr 1994;83(4):412–3.

[32] Gallagher EJ, Rodriguez K, Touger M. Agreement between peripheral venous and arterial lactate levels. Ann Emerg Med 1997;29(4):479–83.

[33] Marshall JC, Vincent JL, Fink MP, et al. Measures, markers, and mediators: toward a staging system for clinical sepsis. A report of the Fifth Toronto Sepsis Roundtable, Toronto, Ontario, Canada, October 25–26, 2000. Crit Care Med 2003;31(5):1560–7.

[34] Simon L, Gauvin F, Amre DK, et al. Serum procalcitonin and c-reactive protein levels as markers of bacterial infection: a systematic review and meta-analysis. Clin Infect Dis 2004; 39(2):206–17 (errata 2005;40:1386–8).

[35] Tang BMP, Eslick GD, McLean AS. Accuracy of procalcitonin for sepsis diagnosis in critically ill patients: a systematic review and meta-analysis. Lancet Infect Dis 2007;7(3):210–7.

[36] Jensen JU, Heslet L, Jensen TH, et al. Procalcitonin increase in early identification of critically ill patients at risk of mortality. Crit Care Med 2006;34(10):2596–602.

[37] Weinstein MP. Current blood culture methods and systems: clinical concepts, technology, and interpretation of results. Clin Infect Dis 1996;23(1):40–6.

[38] Cockerill FR III, Wilson JW, Vetter EA, et al. Optimal testing parameters for blood cultures. Clin Infect Dis 2004;38(12):1724–30.

[39] Mermel LA, Maki DG. Detection of bacteremia in adults: consequences of culturing an inadequate volume of blood. Ann Intern Med 1993;119(4):270–2.

[40] Lamy B, Roy P, Carret G, et al. What is the relevance of obtaining multiple blood samples for culture? A comprehensive model to optimize the strategy for diagnosing bacteremia. Clin Infect Dis 2002;35(7):842–50.

[41] Washington JA II, Ilstrup DM. Blood cultures: issues and controversies. Rev Infect Dis 1986;8(5):792–802.

[42] Aronson MD, Bor DH. Blood cultures. Ann Intern Med 1987;106(2):246–53.

[43] Mandell LA, Wunderink RG, Anzueto A, et al. Infectious Diseases Society of America/American Thoracic Society consensus guidelines on the management of community-acquired pneumonia in adults. Clin Infect Dis 2007;44(Suppl 2):S27–72.

[44] Jones AE, Focht A, Horton JM, et al. Prospective external validation of the clinical effectiveness of an emergency department-based early goal directed therapy protocol for severe sepsis and septic shock. Chest 2007;132(2):425–32.

[45] Nguyen HB, Corbett SW, Steele R, et al. Implementation of a bundle of quality indicators for the early management of severe sepsis and septic shock is associated with decreased mortality. Crit Care Med 2007;35(4):1105–12.

[46] Shorr AF, Micek ST, Jackson WL, et al. Economic implications of an evidence-based sepsis protocol: can we improve outcomes and lower costs? Crit Care Med 2007;35(5):1257–62.

[47] Otari RM, Nguyen HB, Huang DT, et al. Early goal-directed therapy in severe sepsis ands septic shock revisited: concepts, controversies, and contemporary findings. Chest 2006; 130(4):1579–95.

[48] Marik PE, Varon J. Goal-directed therapy for severe sepsis. N Engl J Med 2002;346(13): 1025–6, author reply 1025–6.

[49] Jones AE, Kline JA. Use of goal-directed therapy for severe sepsis and septic shock in academic emergency departments. Crit Care Med 2005;33(8):1888–9.

[50] Shapiro NI, Howell MD, Talmor D, et al. Implementation and outcomes of the Multiple Urgent Sepsis Therapies (MUST) protocol. Crit Care Med 2006;34(4):1025–32.

[51] Micek ST, Roubinian N, Heuring T, et al. Before-after study of a standardized hospital order set for the management of septic shock. Crit Care Med 2006;34(11):2707–13.

[52] Randazzo MR, Snoey ER, Levitt MA. Binder K Accuracy of emergency physician assessment of left ventricular ejection fraction and central venous pressure using echocardiography. Acad Emerg Med 2003;10(9):973–7.

[53] DuPont HL, Spink WW. Infections due to gram-negative organisms: an analysis of 860 patients with bacteremia at the University of Minnesota Medical Center. Medicine 1969; 48(4):307–32.

[54] Freid MA, Vosti KL. The importance of underlying disease in patients with gram-negative bacteremia. Arch Intern Med 1968;121(5):418–23.

[55] Bryant RE, Hood AF, Hood CE, et al. Factors affecting mortality of gram-negative rod bacteremia. Arch Intern Med 1971;127(1):120–8.

[56] Myerowitz RL, Medeiros AA, O'Brien TF. Recent experience with bacillemia due to gram-negative organisms. J Infect Dis 1971;124(3):239–46.

[57] Setia U, Gross PA. Bacteremia in a community hospital: spectrum and mortality. Arch Intern Med 1977;137(12):1698–701.

[58] Weinstein MP, Reller LB, Murphy JR, et al. The clinical significance of positive blood cultures: a comprehensive analysis of 500 episodes of bacteremia and fungemia in adults. I. Laboratory and epidemiologic observations. Rev Infect Dis 1983;5(1):35–53.

[59] Weinstein MP, Murphy JR, Reller LB, et al. The clinical significance of positive blood cultures: a comprehensive analysis of 500 episodes of bacteremia and fungemia in adults. II. Clinical observations, with special reference to factors influencing prognosis. Rev Infect Dis 1983;5(1):54–70.

[60] McCue JD. Improved mortality in gram-negative bacillary bacteremia. Arch Intern Med 1985;145(7):1212–6.

[61] Ispahani P, Pearson NJ, Greenwood D. An analysis of community and hospital-acquired bacteraemia in a large teaching hospital in the United Kingdom. Q J Med 1987;63(241):427–40.

[62] Meyers BR, Sherman E, Mendelson MH, et al. Bloodstream infections in the elderly. Am J Med 1989;86(4):379–84.

[63] Leibovici L, Shraga I, Drucker M, et al. The benefit of appropriate empirical antibiotic treatment in patients with bloodstream infection. J Intern Med 1998;244(5):379–86.

[64] Behrendt G, Schneider S, Brodt HR, et al. Influence of antimicrobial treatment on mortality in septicemia. J Chemother 1999;11(3):179–86.

[65] Zaragoza R, Artero A, Camarena JJ, et al. The influence of inadequate empirical antimicrobial treatment on patients with bloodstream infections in an intensive care unit. Clin Microbiol Infect 2003;9(5):412–8.

[66] Kollef MH, Sherman G, Ward S, et al. Inadequate antimicrobial treatment of infections: a risk factor for hospital mortality among critically ill patients. Chest 1999;115(2):462–74.

[67] Kang CI, Kim SH, Kim HB, et al. Pseudomonas aeruginosa bacteremia: risk factors for mortality and influence of delayed receipt of effective antimicrobial therapy on clinical outcome. Clin Infect Dis 2003;37(6):745–51.

[68] Ibrahim EH, Sherman G, Ward S, et al. The influence of inadequate antimicrobial treatment of bloodstream infections on patient outcomes in the ICU setting. Chest 2000;118(1):146–55.

[69] Yu VL, Chiou CC, Feldman C, et al. An international prospective study of pneumococcal bacteremia: correlation with in vitro resistance, antibiotics administered, and clinical outcome. Clin Infect Dis 2003;37(2):230–7.

[70] Garnacho-Montaro J, Garcia-Garmendia JL, Barrero-Almodovar A, et al. Impact of adequate empirical antibiotic therapy on the outcome of patients admitted to the intensive care unit with sepsis. Crit Care Med 2003;31(12):2742–51.

[71] Valles J, Rello J, Ochagavia A, et al. Community-acquired bloodstream infection in critically ill adult patients: impact of shock and inappropriate antibiotic therapy on survival. Chest 2003;123(5):1615–24.

[72] Cartwright K, Reilly S, White D, et al. Early treatment with parenteral penicillin in meningococcal disease. BMJ 1992;305(6846):143–7.

[73] Kumar A, Roberts D, Wood KE, et al. Duration of hypotension before initiation of effective antimicrobial therapy is the critical determinant of survival in human septic shock. Crit Care Med 2006;34(6):1589–96.

[74] Kumar A, Haery C, Paladugu B, et al. The duration of hypotension before the initiation of antibiotic treatment is a critical determinant of survival in a murine model of *Escherichia*

coli septic shock: association with serum lactate and inflammatory cytokine levels. J Infect Dis 2006;193(2):251–8.

[75] Talan DA, Guterman JJ, Overturf GD, et al. Analysis of the emergency department management of bacterial meningitis. Ann Emerg Med 1989;18(8):856–62.

[76] Aronin SI, Peduzzi P, Quagliarello VJ. Community-acquired bacterial meningitis: risk stratification for adverse clinical outcome and effect of antibiotic timing. Ann Intern Med 1998;129(11):862–9.

[77] Sands KE, Bates DW, Lanken PN, et al. Epidemiology of sepsis syndrome in 8 academic medical centers. Academic Medical Center Consortium Sepsis Project Working Group. JAMA 1997;278(3):234–40.

[78] Brun-Buisson C, Doyon F, Carlet J, et al. Incidence, risk factors, and outcome of severe sepsis and septic shock in adults. A multicenter prospective study in intensive care units. French ICU Group for Severe Sepsis. JAMA 1995;274(12):968–74.

[79] Bochud PY, Glauser MP, Calandra T. Antibiotics in sepsis. Intensive Care Med 2001; 27(Suppl 1):S33–48.

[80] Abraham E, Wunderink R, Silverman H, et al. Efficacy and safety of monoclonal antibody to human tumor necrosis factor alpha in patients with sepsis syndrome. A randomized, controlled, double-blind, multicenter clinical trial. TNF-alpha MAb Sepsis Study Group. JAMA 1995;273(12):934–41.

[81] Brun-Buisson C, Doyon F, Carlet J. Bacteremia and severe sepsis in adults: a multicenter prospective survey in ICUs and wards of 24 hospitals. French Bacteremia-Sepsis Study Group. Am J Respir Crit Care Med 1996;154(3 Pt 1):617–24.

[82] Cohen J, Carlet J. INTERSEPT: an international, multicenter, placebo-controlled trial of monoclonal antibody to human tumor necrosis factor-alpha in patients with sepsis. International Sepsis Trial Study Group. Crit Care Med 1996;24(9):1431–40.

[83] McCabe WR, Jackson GG. Gram negative bacteremia. Arch Intern Med 1962;110:92–100.

[84] Schumer W. Steroids in the treatment of clinical septic shock. Ann Surg 1976;184(3):333–41.

[85] Abraham E, Anzueto A, Gutierrez G, et al. Double-blind randomized controlled trial of monoclonal antibody to human tumour necrosis factor in treatment of septic shock. NORASEPT II Study Group. Lancet 1998;351(9107):929–33.

[86] Saravolatz LD, Wherry JC, Spooner C, et al. Clinical safety, tolerability, and pharmacokinetics of murine monoclonal antibody to human tumor necrosis factor-alpha. J Infect Dis 1994;169(1):214–7.

[87] Kieft H, Hoepelman AI, Zhou W, et al. The sepsis syndrome in a Dutch university hospital. Clinical observations. Arch Intern Med 1993;153(19):2241–7.

[88] Fisher CJ Jr, Dhainaut JF, Opal SM, et al. Recombinant human interleukin 1 receptor antagonist in the treatment of patients with sepsis syndrome. Results from a randomized, double-blind, placebo-controlled trial. Phase III rhIL-1ra Sepsis Syndrome Study Group. JAMA 1994;271(23):1836–43.

[89] Fisher CJ Jr, Slotman GJ, Opal SM, et al. Initial evaluation of human recombinant interleukin-1 receptor antagonist in the treatment of sepsis syndrome: a randomized, open-label, placebo-controlled multicenter trial. The IL-1RA Sepsis Syndrome Study Group. Crit Care Med 1994;22(1):12–21.

[90] Reinhart K, Wiegand-Lohnert C, Grimminger F, et al. Assessment of the safety and efficacy of the monoclonal anti-tumor necrosis factor antibody-fragment, MAK 195F, in patients with sepsis and septic shock: a multicenter, randomized, placebo-controlled, dose-ranging study. Crit Care Med 1996;24(5):733–42.

[91] Dhainaut JF, Vincent JL, Richard C, et al. CDP571, a humanized antibody to human tumor necrosis factor-alpha: safety, pharmacokinetics, immune response, and influence of the antibody on cytokine concentrations in patients with septic shock. CPD571 Sepsis Study Group. Crit Care Med 1995;23(9):1461–9.

[92] Opal SM, Fisher CJ Jr, Dhainaut JF, et al. Confirmatory interleukin-1 receptor antagonist trial in severe sepsis: a phase III, randomized, double-blind, placebo-controlled, multicenter trial. The Interleukin-1 Receptor Antagonist Sepsis Investigator Group. Crit Care Med 1997;25(7):1115–24.

[93] Bernard GR, Wheeler AP, Russell JA, et al. The effects of ibuprofen on the physiology and survival of patients with sepsis. The Ibuprofen in Sepsis Study Group. N Engl J Med 1997; 336(13):912–8.

[94] Mylotte JM, Tayara A, Goodnough S. Epidemiology of bloodstream infection in nursing home residents: evaluation in a large cohort from multiple homes. Clin Infect Dis 2002; 35(12):1484–90.

[95] Osih RB, McGregor JC, Rich SE, et al. Impact of empiric antibiotic therapy on outcomes in patients with Pseudomonas aeruginosa bacteremia. Antimicrob Agents Chemother 2007; 51(13):839–44.

[96] Vanderkooi OG, Low DE, Green K, et al. Toronto Invasive Bacterial Disease Network. Predicting antimicrobial resistance in invasive pneumococcal infections. Clin Infect Dis 2005;40(9):1288–97.

[97] Wenzel RP, Sahm DF, Thornsberry C, et al. In vitro susceptibilities of gram-negative bacteria isolated from hospitalized patients in four European countries, Canada, and the United States in 2000–2001 to expanded-spectrum cephalosporins and comparator antimicrobials: implications for therapy. Antimicrob Agents Chemother 2003;47(10): 3089–98.

[98] Karlowsky JA, Jones ME, Thornsberry C, et al. Stable antimicrobial susceptibility rates for clinical isolates of Pseudomonas aeruginosa from the 2001–2003 tracking resistance in the United States today surveillance studies. Clin Infect Dis 2005;40(Suppl 2): S89–98.

[99] Karlowsky JA, Thornsberry C, Critchley IA, et al. Susceptibilities to levofloxacin in Streptococcus pneumoniae, Haemophilus influenzae, and Moraxella catarrhalis clinical isolates from children: results from 2000–2001 and 2001–2002 TRUST studies in the United States. Antimicrob Agents Chemother 2003;47(6):1790–7.

[100] Draghi DC, Sheehan DJ, Hogan P, et al. In vitro activity of linezolid against key gram-positive organisms isolated in the United States: results of the LEADER 2004 surveillance program. Antimicrob Agents Chemother 2005;49(12):5024–32.

[101] Chen DK, McGeer A, de Azavedo JC, et al. Decreased susceptibility of Streptococcus pneumoniae to fluoroquinolones in Canada. Canadian Bacterial Surveillance Network. N Engl J Med 1999;341(4):233–9.

[102] Moran GJ, Krishnadasan A, Gorwitz RJ, et al, for The EMERGEncy ID NET Study Group. Methicillin-resistant S. aureus infections among patients in the emergency department. N Engl J Med 2006;355(7):666–74.

[103] Centers for Disease Control. Severe methicillin-resistant Staphylococcus aureus community-nity-acquired pneumonia associated with influenza–Louisiana and Georgia, December 2006–January 2007. MMWR Morb Mortal Wkly Rep 2007;56(14):325–9.

[104] Ruhe JJ, Smith N, Bradsher RW, et al. Community-onset methicillin-resistant Staphylococcus aureus skin and soft-tissue infections: impact of antimicrobial therapy on outcome. Clin Infect Dis 2007;44(6):777–84.

[105] Szumowski JD, Cohen DE, Kanaya F, et al. Treatment and outcomes of infections by methicillin-resistant Staphylococcus aureus at an ambulatory clinic. Antimicrob Agents Chemother 2007;51(2):423–8.

[106] Dragi DC, Sheehan DF, Hogan P, et al. Current antimicrobial resistance profiles among methicillin-resistant Staphylococcus aureus encountered in the outpatient setting. Diagn Microbiol Infect Dis 2006;55(2):129–33.

[107] Lewis JS II, Jorgensen JH. Inducible clindamycin resistance in Staphylococci: should clinicians and microbiologists be concerned? Clin Infect Dis 2005;40(2):280–5.

[108] Centers for Disease Control. Invasive methicillin-resistant *Staphylococcus aureus* infections among dialysis patients—United States, 2005. MMWR Morb Mortal Wkly Rep 2007; 56(9):197–9.

[109] Deresinski S. Counterpoint: Vancomycin and *Staphylococcus aureus*–an antibiotic enters obsolescence. Clin Infect Dis 2007;44(12):1543–8.

[110] Mohr JF, Murray BE. Point: Vancomycin is not obsolete for the treatment of infection caused by methicillin-resistant *Staphylococcus aureus*. Clin Infect Dis 2007;44(12):1536–42.

[111] Lodise TP Jr, McKinnon PS, Levine DP, et al. Impact of empirical therapy selection on outcomes of intravenous drug users with infective endocarditis caused by methicillin susceptible *Staphylococcus aureus*. Antimicrob Agents Chemother 2007;51(10):3731–3.

[112] Stevens DL, Ma Y, Salmi DB, et al. Impact of antibiotics on expression of virulence-associated exotoxin genes in methicillin-sensitive and methicillin-resistant *Staphylococcus aureus*. J Infect Dis 2007;195(2):202–11.

[113] Harbarth S, Nobre V, Pittet D. Does antibiotic selection impact patient outcome? Clin Infect Dis 2007;44(1):87–93.

[114] Hunter TH. Use of streptomycin in treatment of bacterial endocarditis. Am J Med 1947;2: 436–42.

[115] Fowler VG Jr, Boucher HW, Corey GR, et al. Paptomycin versus standard therapy for bacteremia and endocarditis caused by *Staphylococcus aureus*. N Engl J Med 2006;355(7): 653–5.

[116] Howden BP, Ward PB, Charles PGP, et al. Treatment outcomes for serious infections caused by methicillin-resistant *Staphylococcus aureus* with reduced vancomycin susceptibility. Clin Infect Dis 2004;38(4):521–8.

[117] Weigelt J, Itani K, Stevens D, et al, and the Linezolid CSSTI Study Group. Linezolid versus vancomycin in treatment of complicated skin and soft tissue infections. Antimicrob Agents Chemother 2005;49(6):2260–6.

[118] Wunderink RG, Rello J, Cammarata SK, et al. Linezolid vs vancomycin: analysis of two double-blind studies of patients with methicillin-resistant *Staphylococcus aureus* nosocomial pneumonia. Chest 2003;124(5):1789–97.

[119] Jensen AG, Wachmann CH, Espersen F, et al. Treatment and outcome of *Staphylococcus aureus* bacteremia: a prospective study of 278 cases. Arch Intern Med 2002;162(1):25–32.

[120] Bohnen JM, Marshall JC, Fry DE, et al. Clinical and scientific importance of source control in abdominal infections: summary of a symposium. Can J Surg 1999;42(2):122–6.

[121] Knaus WA, Draper EA, Wagner DP, et al. APACHE II: a severity of disease classification system. Crit Care Med 1985;13(10):818–29.

[122] FDA briefing document. Drotrecogin alfa (activated) [recombinant human activated protein C (rhAPC)] Xigris, BLA#125029/0. Food and Drug Administration. Available at: www.fda.gov/ohrms/dockets/ac/01/briefing/3797b1.htm. Accessed September 12, 2001.

[123] Abraham EA, LaTerre PF, Garg R, et al. Drotrecogin alfa (activated) for adults with severe sepsis and a low risk of death. N Engl J Med 2005;353(123):1332–41.

[124] Nadel S, Goldstein B, Williams MD, et al. Drotrecogin alfa (activated) in children with severe sepsis: a multicentre phase III randomized controlled trial. Lancet 2007;369(9564): 836–43.

[125] Ely EW, Bernard GR, Vincent JL. Activated protein C for severe sepsis. N Engl J Med 2002;347(13):1035–6.

[126] Vincent JL, Bernard GR, Beale R, et al. Drotrecogin alfa (activated) treatment in severe sepsis from the global open-label trial ENHANCE: further evidence for survival and safety and implications for early treatment. Crit Care Med 2005;33(10):2266–77.

[127] Vincent J-L, O'Brien JO Jr, Wheeler A, et al. Use of an integrated clinical trial database to evaluate the effect of timing of drotrecogin alfa (activated) treatment in severe sepsis. Crit Care 2006;10(3):R74.

[128] Warren HS, Suffredini AF, Eichacker PQ, et al. Risks and benefits of activated protein C treatment for severe sepsis. N Engl J Med 2002;347(13):1027–30.

[129] Laterre P-F, Garber G, Levy H, et al. Severe community-acquired pneumonia as a cause of severe sepsis: Data from the PROWESS study. Crit Care Med 2005;33(5):952–61.

[130] Haley M, Cui X, Minneci PC, et al. Recombinant human activated protein C in sepsis: Previous concerns and current usage. Therapy 2004;1:123–9.

[131] Lilly Plans New Clinical Trial Of Xigris(R). Available at: http://www.medicalnewstoday.com/articles/63959.php. Accessed August 20, 2007.

[132] Annane D, Sebille V, Troche G, et al. A 3-level prognostic classification in septic shock based on cortisol levels and cortisol response to corticotropin. JAMA 2000;283(8):1038–45.

[133] Lamberts SW, Bruining HA, de Jong FH. Corticosteroid therapy in severe illness. N Engl J Med 1997;337(18):1285–92.

[134] Sprung CL, Caralis PV, Marcial EH, et al. The effects of high-dose corticosteroids in patients with septic shock: a prospective, controlled study. N Engl J Med 1984;311(18):1137–43.

[135] Bone RC, Fisher CJ Jr, Clemmer TP, et al. A controlled clinical trial of high-dose methylprednisolone in the treatment of severe sepsis and septic shock. N Engl J Med 1987;317(11):653–8.

[136] The Veterans Administration Systemic Sepsis Cooperative Study Group. Effect of high-dose glucocorticoid therapy on mortality in patients with clinical signs of systemic sepsis. N Engl J Med 1987;317(11):659–65.

[137] Annane D, Sebille V, Charpentier C, et al. Effect of treatment with low doses of hydrocortisone and fludrocortisone on mortality in patients with septic shock. JAMA 2002;288(7):862–71.

[138] Sprung CL, Annane D, Briegel J, et al. Hydrocortisone therapy for patients with septic shock. N Eng J Med 2008;358(2):111–24.

[139] Ventilation with lower tidal volumes as compared with traditional tidal volumes for acute lung injury and the acute respiratory distress syndrome. The Acute Respiratory Distress Syndrome Network. N Engl J Med 2000;342(18):1301–8.

[140] Van den Berghe G, Wouters P, Weekers F, et al. Intensive insulin therapy in the critically ill patients. N Engl J Med 2001;345(19):1359–67.

[141] Van den Berghe G, Wilmer A, Hermans G, et al. Intensive insulin therapy in the medical ICU. N Engl J Med 2006;354(5):449–61.

[142] Cooper DJ, Walley KR, Wiggs BR, et al. Bicarbonate does not improve hemodynamics in critically ill patients who have lactic acidosis. A prospective, controlled clinical study. Ann Intern Med 1990;112(3):492–8.

[143] Mathieu D, Neviere R, Billard V, et al. Effects of bicarbonate therapy on hemodynamics and tissue oxygenation in patients with lactic acidosis: a prospective, controlled clinical study. Crit Care Med 1991;19(11):1352–6.

ELSEVIER
SAUNDERS

Infect Dis Clin N Am 22 (2008) 33–52

INFECTIOUS
DISEASE CLINICS
OF NORTH AMERICA

Emergency Department Management of Meningitis and Encephalitis

Michael T. Fitch, MD, PhD, FACEP, FAAEM[a],*,
Fredrick M. Abrahamian, DO, FACEP[b,c],
Gregory J. Moran, MD, FACEP, FAAEM[b,c,d],
David A. Talan, MD, FACEP, FAAEM, FIDSA[b,c,d]

[a]Department of Emergency Medicine, Wake Forest University School of Medicine,
Medical Center Boulevard, Winston-Salem, NC 27157, USA
[b]David Geffen School of Medicine at University of California Los Angeles,
Los Angeles, CA, USA
[c]Department of Emergency Medicine, Olive View-University of California Los Angeles
Medical Center, 14445 Olive View Drive, North Annex, Sylmar, CA 91342-1438, USA
[d]Department of Medicine, Division of Infectious Diseases, Olive View-University of California
Los Angeles Medical Center, 1445 Olive View Drive, North Annex,
Sylmar, CA 91342-1438, USA

Bacterial meningitis and viral encephalitis are infectious disease emergencies that can cause significant patient morbidity and mortality. Controversies remain about accuracy of clinical evaluation, role of radiographic imaging before lumbar puncture (LP), interpretation of cerebrospinal fluid (CSF) analysis, and standards for timely antibiotic administration [1]. With an estimated incidence of 2.6 to 6 per 100,000 adults per year in developed countries [2–5], bacterial meningitis continues to have mortality rates of 13% to 27% [4,6–11]. Although serious morbidity is rare with viral meningitis [12,13], acute herpes simplex virus (HSV) encephalitis has a mortality rate of 20% to 50% with appropriate therapy [14,15]. With the advent of *Haemophilus influenzae* type b and conjugate pneumococcal vaccines, and the recently expanded recommendations for use of conjugated meningococcal vaccine, the incidence of bacterial meningitis has decreased compared with that of the prevaccine era and relative to the large numbers of patients with fever and headache owing to other causes. Whereas the infectious

Dr. Fitch received faculty funding support for his work on this project from the Brooks Scholars in Academic Medicine award at the Wake Forest University School of Medicine.

* Corresponding author.

E-mail address: mfitch@wfubmc.edu (M.T. Fitch).

diseases specialist is often involved when such diagnoses are highly suspected or confirmed, emergency physicians are challenged to identify these cases among a broad population of patients with undifferentiated complaints.

Emergency clinicians need to accurately diagnose patients and administer timely antimicrobials and adjunctive therapies to those patients who need them while attempting to avoid unnecessary, time-consuming, and invasive testing and treatment of patients without these diseases. Among the most common and costly malpractice lawsuits are those for patients diagnosed with meningitis who subsequently had poor clinical outcomes [16]. This article focuses on the identification of patients with bacterial meningitis from the perspective of the emergency physician, and discusses HSV as another important and treatable cause of acute central nervous system (CNS) infection. The frequency of historical and physical examination findings among patients with bacterial meningitis, interpretation of CSF results, issues related to the timeliness of treatment, and specific recommendations for antimicrobials and corticosteroids are also presented.

History and physical exam to diagnose central nervous system infections

Clinical suspicion of a CNS infection begins with patient history. Conditions that may increase a patient's risk of contracting an infection, such as asplenia or CNS prosthetic device, should be initially considered along with epidemiologic factors (eg, a household contact of an index meningococcal infection case, or a newborn in the setting of maternal genital herpes) when assessing risk. Nonspecific symptoms such as headache, nausea, and vomiting are poor predictors of meningitis [17], which is not surprising considering the large numbers of patients with these nonspecific complaints who are evaluated in the emergency department (ED). Large series of patients with bacterial meningitis provide information about aspects of patient history that are associated with this CNS infection. However, these are of limited usefulness as the performance characteristics of these findings have not been studied in undifferentiated ED populations. It is notable that in one study, the historical "classic triad" of fever, stiff neck, and altered mental status was found in only two thirds of 493 episodes of bacterial meningitis in adults. At least one of the elements of the triad was found in all patients, and the nonspecific finding of fever was the most common feature [3]. Other studies among adults with bacterial meningitis found somewhat lower proportions of patients (51%) with this classic triad of symptoms [11], or symptoms of fever, stiff neck, and headache (66%) [9]. A study that pooled results of 11 studies involving 845 patients found that the classic triad was found in 46% of patients with meningitis, but 99% had at least one feature [17]. A more recent study of 696 episodes of bacterial meningitis in adults from the Netherlands reported the classic triad of symptoms in less than 50% and fever in only 77% of patients. At least two of four elements (headache, fever, neck stiffness, and altered mental status) were present in 95% of patients in this study [4]. These findings illustrate the difficulty faced by emergency physicians as many cases of bacterial meningitis lack the typical constellation of findings that would help to distinguish this infrequent life-threatening diagnosis from more common and benign conditions. In addition, some common aspects of history may be more difficult or impossible to obtain in young children who cannot verbalize complaints such as headache and neck stiffness.

Although meningitis should be considered in the differential diagnosis of children who present with febrile seizure, it is not necessary to perform LP in most cases of well- appearing children with normal mental status. One retrospective study of more than 500 children with meningitis found that, although 23% had seizures on presentation, in no case was seizure the sole manifestation of bacterial meningitis [18]. All cases had other findings that suggested meningitis, such as persistent altered mental status, nuchal rigidity, or multiple seizures. Children older than 2 months with a simple febrile seizure whose mental status clears quickly and who have no other signs of CNS infection can be safely discharged home on antipyretics without an LP after an age-appropriate workup for the febrile illness.

Physical examination is an important next step in the evaluation of patients in whom the history has suggested the possibility of a CNS infection. Neck stiffness, altered mental status, and fever are all clinical findings that are often used in a clinician's evaluation for possible meningitis. However, several studies have suggested that these signs are inadequately sensitive to identify patients with meningitis or encephalitis. One meta-analysis found that the presence of a documented fever had a sensitivity of only 85%, whereas examination findings of neck stiffness and altered mental status had sensitivities of 70% and 67%, respectively [17]. This meta-analysis also found that meningitis was unlikely when fever, neck stiffness, and altered mental status were all absent. Neck stiffness is found in 60% to 70% of pediatric patients with bacterial or viral meningitis [19–21], although this finding may be less commonly found in children younger than 1 year [19].

Classically described meningeal findings such as Kernig's sign (flexing the hip and extending the knee to elicit pain in the back and legs), Brudzinski's sign (passive flexion of the neck elicits flexion of the hips), and nuchal rigidity (severe neck stiffness) have been found in prospective studies of adults with meningitis (defined by CSF pleocytosis) to have sensitivities of only 5% to 30% [22,23]. It is unclear whether these findings are more frequently present in bacterial meningitis. A small prospective study of 54 patients with meningitis found that jolt accentuation (exacerbation of an existing headache with rapid head rotation) had a sensitivity of 97%, but this clinical test has not been evaluated in any subsequent larger studies [23].

The clinical presentation of patients with encephalitis can be similar to patients with meningitis, but no large series of patients with encephalitis exist to clearly define the frequency of specific features. Although many of the presenting signs and symptoms are the same, encephalitis is suggested by the presence of altered mental status and focal neurologic findings [24].

Clinicians should also be aware that patients with bacterial meningitis may have presentations consistent with encephalitis owing to complications such as cerebral edema and stroke.

Is central nervous system imaging required before lumbar puncture?

LP is indicated in patients in whom bacterial meningitis or encephalitis is suspected after history and physical examination is completed. LP is associated with common minor side effects such as post-LP headaches, local back pain, and bleeding from the spinal needle insertion. One more serious complication that has been discussed since the first LPs were performed in the late 1800s is brain herniation. CT scan of the head is used to identify patients at higher risk for herniation with intracranial pathology such as hydrocephalus, mass lesions, cerebral edema, and midline brain shift. The indications for obtaining a CT scan of the head before LP are at present debated.

That LP may precipitate brain herniation is based on case reports suggesting a temporal relationship [25–27]. The issue remains unclear, however, as patients with meningitis can have brain herniation without undergoing LP, and other patients may have normal CT scans and subsequently suffer herniation [25,26,28]. One review of 200 LPs in patients with increased intracranial pressure (ICP) from brain tumors reported no adverse effects of this procedure [29], a finding supported by another series in which LP was performed in 103 patients with increased ICP and only four complications were observed [30]. Even patients with papilledema have had LP done without apparent complications [29,31,32], and LP is therapeutic in patients with increased ICP owing to pseudotumor cerebri. Herniation from LP requires both increased ICP and obstruction to free CSF flow and equilibration [33].

CT scan of the head can be used to help identify patients with lesions that place them at risk of herniation from LP, and to diagnose conditions that would make LP unnecessary or that would be missed if the patient's workup was limited to LP (eg, tumors and abscesses). One set of recommendations for CT scanning before LP is based on one single-center prospective study of adults with suspected meningitis that has yet to be validated [34]. This study associated an abnormal CT scan with the following characteristics: age greater than 60, seizure in the past 1 week, immunocompromise, history of CNS disease, altered mental status, gaze or facial palsy, abnormal language or inability to answer two questions or follow two commands, visual field abnormalities, and arm or leg drift. It has been recommended that CT of the head is unnecessary before LP if these findings are absent, thus reducing evaluation times, costs, and patient radiation exposure. However, for the small group without these risk factors (96 patients; 41% of enrolled patients), the frequency of an abnormal CT scan was 3%, with an upper limit of the 95% CI of 9%. This suggests the possibility of an abnormal CT in 1 of 11 patients tested.

Decision rules like this one may not identify all patients with an intracranial lesion, as patients with headache and fever from a brain abscess do not consistently have focal neurologic findings, such as for lesions in the frontal lobe [35]. CSF pleocytosis associated with a parameningeal focus from an intracranial abscess could be confused with meningitis if CNS imaging were not obtained. Many ED patients with HIV/AIDS are unaware of their HIV infection and may be at risk for toxoplasmosis or CNS lymphoma that could be diagnosed by CT scan. In general, children are at lower risk than adults for these kinds of alternative CNS diagnoses, and CT scanning may have less of a role in this population if risk factors are absent. The decision to first obtain CT imaging before LP also should not affect the decision to initiate critical therapies such as antibiotics and corticosteroids, as is discussed below.

When assessing for possible risks of herniation, obtaining CT scanning of the head is recommended before LP for those patients with high-risk features such as new-onset seizures, immunocompromise, papilledema, focal neurologic signs, or impaired consciousness [1]. CT scan is indicated for diagnostic purposes in patients with risk factors for intracranial lesions such as brain abscess (eg, concurrent head and neck infection) or malignancy, and should be considered for patients who cannot provide a good history or who have not had past medical evaluation. CT scan may also be useful after LP results are available—for example, to evaluate the finding of increased intracranial pressure. Patients with encephalitis will usually have indications for initial CT imaging, and HSV encephalitis has characteristic temporal lobe abnormalities. Although MRI with contrast appears to be more sensitive for detection of these findings, it is of less utility initially because of lack of availability and the longer time required to complete the study compared with CT scan.

Cerebrospinal fluid results—can viral and bacterial disease be distinguished?

Cerebrospinal fluid cytology and chemistry studies

Once LP is successfully completed, CSF analysis will help the clinician to make the diagnosis of meningitis or encephalitis on the basis of increased CSF white blood cell (WBC) counts. Typical CSF findings for viral CNS infection include WBC counts fewer than 300 cells per mm^3, less than 20% of which are neutrophils, and normal protein and glucose levels. HSV encephalitis is characterized by temporal lobe hemorrhage, edema, and necrosis with inflammation, which, in addition to CSF lymphocytic pleocytosis, can be accompanied by increased CSF red blood cells [15,24,36,37]. In the absence of a positive Gram stain, bacterial meningitis is more likely with CSF WBC counts greater than 1000 cells per mm^3, greater than 80% of which are neutrophils, and elevated protein and reduced glucose levels.

However, these typical findings do not allow the correct diagnosis of all patients, as bacterial meningitis has been described in patients with fewer than 100 cells per mm^3 in the CSF [3,4,6,9,11], and, in one study of 696 episodes of bacterial meningitis, 12% of patients had none of the CSF findings characteristic of bacterial etiology [4]. On the other hand, 30% to 50% of patients with viral meningitis have a CSF neutrophil predominance, a finding typically described in bacterial disease [20,38,39]. Although oral or intravenous antibiotics given before LP will decrease the yield of CSF gram stain and cultures in cases of bacterial meningitis, CSF cytochemical abnormalities are not readily affected [40–42]. The yield of gram stain in cases of bacterial meningitis is 50% to 90% [3,4,40,41,43], but decreases 7% to 41% among patients taking oral antibiotics [40].

Many studies of children with meningitis have developed scoring systems to help clinicians to predict the risk of bacterial disease [44–49]. The Bacterial Meningitis Score [49] is one of these systems that has been recently validated in a multicenter retrospective cohort study of 2903 children with CSF pleocytosis. In the study, 121 (4.2%) were found to have bacterial meningitis and the absence of all five variables (one point each) included in the scoring system (ie, positive Gram stain, CSF WBC ≥ 1000 cells/μl, CSF protein ≥ 80 mg/dL, peripheral blood absolute neutrophil count ≥ 10,000 cells/μl, and history of seizure before presentation) had a negative predictive value for bacterial meningitis of 99.9%. A score of 1 or more identified all children older than 2 months with this disease. Other scoring systems have been derived [50–54]; however, it is clear that no model is 100% accurate and there is no single variable that can reliably exclude bacterial meningitis when an elevated CSF WBC is found [13,44,48,51,53,55–60]. A prospective multicenter study of 151 adults with CSF pleocytosis and a gram-negative stain found that emergency physician judgment had 89% sensitivity and 77% specificity for the diagnosis of bacterial meningitis and performed with better accuracy than CSF leukocyte count, CSF protein, CSF/blood glucose ratio, percentage of CSF leukocytes, and serum C-reactive protein (CRP) levels [58]. Using the same data set, a comparison of multiple scoring systems found that none were perfect and they appeared to work better in pediatric patients than in adults. Such systems may be useful to help with clinical management but not as exact rules for therapeutic decision making in individual patients [60].

The information from scoring systems and studies that have identified predictors for bacterial disease may be helpful as a supplement to physician judgment, even if they cannot be rigorously applied as decision rules for individual patients. Consideration of Bayes' theorem has been applied to the interpretation of CSF studies [61], and the pretest probability of bacterial meningitis can significantly impact the posttest probability of disease when examining the performance characteristics of CSF findings such as the cell count and differential. For example, in a young immunocompetent patient who presents during summer months in the midst of a known enteroviral outbreak with signs and symptoms of viral disease (ie, a low pretest probability for bacterial meningitis), CSF findings not suggestive of bacterial infection would lead to a very low posttest probability of bacterial disease such that hospital admission for empiric antibiotic therapy would not be required. On the other hand, severely ill patients (eg, with hypotension or altered mental status) or significant risk factors (eg, sickle cell anemia with functional asplenia) have a higher pretest probability of bacterial meningitis. Even if CSF findings are suggestive of viral meningitis, the posttest probability of bacterial disease may still be significantly high such that empiric antibiotic treatment and hospital admission would be indicated.

Other laboratory investigations

Latex agglutination antigen tests can help to identify bacterial pathogens in the CSF. A wide range of sensitivities (50%–100%) have been reported for detection of the most common bacterial causes of meningitis, and therefore a negative result alone does not allow exclusion of bacterial meningitis, and results may not be available within the time frame of ED care [62]. Some studies find that this testing does not frequently change clinical decisions about antibiotic therapy [63,64], suggesting that it should not be recommended for routine use. This testing method may be most useful for patients with CSF pleocytosis and a gram-negative CSF stain who were treated with antibiotics before LP.

CRP is an acute-phase reactant that has been used as a nonspecific marker of inflammation for many clinical conditions, and some studies have suggested that it may have a role in the diagnosis of bacterial meningitis. A meta-analysis found that, although elevated CRP levels in serum or CSF were associated with increased risk for bacterial meningitis compared with aseptic meningitis, the tests appear to be sensitive but nonspecific, and only a negative test was potentially helpful in clinical settings [65]. Studies published since this analysis have also found an association of higher CRP levels in the serum or CSF with bacterial meningitis [66–68]. Currently, because of limited data from studies with small numbers of patients, and variable methodologies and abnormality thresholds, the clinical utility of this test, which is not consistently available or available within the time frame of ED care, is unclear.

Elevated serum procalcitonin levels have been identified in patients with acute bacterial infections [69], and studies in children and adults suggested a possible role in differentiating bacterial and viral meningitis [68,70–72]. Several small series found high specificity for bacterial meningitis but with limited sensitivity [66,73]. Inconsistent results, and limitations similar to CRP as noted above, have led some to conclude that this test should not be relied on to make individual patient treatment decisions [74].

Viral testing using polymerase chain reaction (PCR) technology is another diagnostic modality that could play a central role to identify patients with aseptic meningitis, and this would be a potentially useful adjunctive test in the ED for CSF samples with pleocytosis. As the most common causes of viral meningitis, enteroviruses are a logical choice for this diagnostic technology. Recent approval by the US Food and Drug Administration of a rapid (ie, less than 3 hours) qualitative test for enteroviral RNA in CSF may facilitate disposition decisions and decrease unnecessary antibiotic therapy and hospitalization. A report of a multicenter trial of this rapid enteroviral assay system found a sensitivity of 97% and specificity of 100% using 102 CSF samples from patients with suspected meningitis [75]. If encephalitis is a consideration, CSF should be sent for HSV PCR, although this study is not available as a rapid test. Other serum and CSF studies for viral encephalitis (eg, West Nile virus serology) would be considered based on the patient's specific risk, epidemiology, and local public health department recommendations.

Causes of meningitis and encephalitis

Bacterial meningitis

Bacterial meningitis in developed countries is estimated to occur in 2.6 to 6 per 100,000 adults per year, and can be many times higher in some undeveloped countries [2–5]. The most common pathogens causing meningitis are *Streptococcus pneumoniae* and *Neisseria meningitidis* [2,4,6]. The median age of patients with meningitis in the United States went up from 15 months in 1986 (before the introduction of the *H influenzae* type b vaccination) to 25 years in 1995 [2]. Childhood vaccination programs for *H influenzae* type b and *S pneumoniae* have thus reduced the incidence of infections due to these pathogens [76,77]; with the recent introduction of a vaccination for *N meningitidis*, it is hoped that the incidence of this infection will also decrease. *Listeria monocytogenes* is a cause of meningitis that is more common in patient groups with specific risk factors such as neonates or adults older than 50, immunocompromise, alcohol abuse, and pregnancy [78].

Aseptic meningitis

By definition, aseptic meningitis is any meningeal irritation in the absence of bacterial infection. Enterovirus infections, such as coxsackie and echoviruses, comprise more than 80% of all episodes of aseptic meningitis and are the most commonly identified causes of CNS viral infections [48,79,80]. HSV is another frequent cause of viral meningitis [81,82], with other viral causes such as mumps, HIV, cytomegalovirus, and varicella-zoster virus being less commonly found in immunocompetent patients. Other infectious causes of aseptic meningitis include organisms that do not grow on routine culture plates such as *Mycobacterium tuberculosis*; *Treponema pallidum*; *Chlamydia* sp; *Mycoplasma* sp; *Rickettsia* sp; and opportunistic fungi such as *Cryptococcus* sp, *Coccidioides* sp, and *Histoplasma* sp [83]. Aseptic meningitis can also be caused by non-infectious causes. Drugs such as ibuprofen [84,85] and trimethoprim-sulfamethoxazole [86] have been implicated. Rheumatologic disorders, such as Sjogren's syndrome, can cause meningitis [87], and there have been reports of meningitis associated with immunizations such as the measle-mumps-rubella vaccine [88]. Although aseptic meningitis is most often caused by viral infection with a typically benign course, clinicians must be careful to also consider the uncommon but treatable causes of meningitis as mentioned above. A description of epidemiologic risk factors and clinical and laboratory findings that would suggest these other diagnoses is beyond the scope of this article, but the overlapping findings with common enteroviral syndromes argue for careful patient education and follow-up.

Viral encephalitis

Viral CNS infection causing life-threatening encephalitis can be distinguished from the typically benign viral meningitis by the presence of altered mental status and/or focal neurologic findings. HSV encephalitis occurs in approximately 1 to 4 per 1,000,000 people per year and is a common cause of fatal CNS infections [12,15,37,89]. HSV-1 causes more than 90% of HSV encephalitis cases; the remainder are caused by HSV-2 [90].

Pharmacologic therapy to treat central nervous system infections

Empiric antibiotics for bacterial meningitis

Bacterial meningitis is a life-threatening infection, and empiric administration of broad-spectrum antibiotics (Table 1) is indicated for patients suffering from this disease until bacterial identification is made [1,5,62,78,91]. Third-generation cephalosporins ceftriaxone and cefotaxime have excellent CSF penetration, provide coverage for the most common bacterial pathogens (including *N meningitidis* and *S pneumoniae*), and are recommended for initial therapy [92]. Vancomycin should be added for coverage of *S pneumoniae* resistant to these third-generation cephalosporins, as the prevalence of resistant isolates or those with intermediate sensitivity to ceftriaxone is as high as 3% in adult patients and 9% in children [93,94]. Patients who abuse alcohol or are immunocompromised, pregnant, a neonate, or older than 50 should also be treated with ampicillin to cover for *L monocytogenes* infection [1,4,5,62,91]. For patients who have a serious penicillin/cephalosporin allergy, chloramphenicol can be substituted for a third-generation cephalosporin and trimethoprim/sulfamethoxazole can be substituted for ampicillin (to treat *L monocytogenes*). As in clinical practice a gradient of risk exists for bacterial meningitis, the addition of other antibiotics to ceftriaxone or cefotaxime, such as vancomycin and ampicillin, and administration of

Table 1
Recommended empiric therapy for adults and children with suspected bacterial meningitis or
herpes simplex virus encephalitis

Patient age	Intravenous empiric therapy[a]
Children[b] 1 mo to 17 y	Dexamethasone, 0.6 mg/kg/d divided every 6 h for 4 d (given before or with first dose of antibiotics)
	Ceftriaxone, 80–100 mg/kg/d divided every 12–24 h, *or* cefotaxime, 225–300 mg/kg/d divided every 6–8 h
	Vancomycin, 60 mg/kg/d divided every 6 h
	Acyclovir, 10 mg/kg given every 8 h, if HSV encephalitis is suspected (may use up to 20 mg/kg every 8 h for children under age 12)
Adults[b] 18–49 y	Dexamethasone, 10 mg given every 6 h for 4 d (given before or with first dose of antibiotics)
	Ceftriaxone, 4 g/d divided every 12–24 h, *or* cefotaxime 8–12 g/d divided every 4–6 h
	Vancomycin, 30–45 mg/kg divided every 8–12 h
	Acyclovir, 10 mg/kg given every 8 h, if HSV encephalitis is suspected
Adults 50 y or older	Dexamethasone, 10 mg given every 6 h for 4 d (given before or with first dose of antibiotics)
	Ceftriaxone, 4 g/d divided every 12–24 h, *or* cefotaxime, 8–12 g/d divided every 4–6 h
	Vancomycin, 30–45 mg/kg divided every 8–12 h
	Ampicillin, 12 g/d divided every 4 h
	Acyclovir, 10 mg/kg given every 8 h, if HSV encephalitis is suspected

Severe penicillin allergy. Can replace third-generation cephalosporin with chloramphenicol (75–100 mg/kg/d divided every 6 h for children; 4–6 g/d divided every 6 h for adults) and can replace ampicillin with trimethoprim-sulfamethoxazole (1–20 mg/kg/d divided every 6–12 h for children and adults).

[a] Antibiotic dosing based on guidelines established by the Infectious Disease Society of America and assumes average weights for age and normal hepatic and renal function, see [62].

[b] Consider additional coverage with ampicillin in patients with risk factors for Listeria such as age older than 50, alcohol abuse, immunocompromise, or pregnancy.

a preceding dose of corticosteroid (as is discussed below), depends on the physician's clinical suspicion of disease.

The Infectious Disease Society of America (IDSA) guidelines state that, "there are inadequate data to delineate specific guidelines on the interval between the initial physician encounter and the administration of the first dose of antimicrobial therapy ..." and "appropriate therapy ... should be initiated as soon as possible after the diagnosis is considered to be likely" [62]. Observational studies in various practice environments have demonstrated that, for patients admitted with the presumptive diagnosis of bacterial meningitis, the average time from ED registration to antibiotic initiation is 3 to 5 hours [7,8,40,95,96]. These findings illustrate the amount of time required for diagnostic evaluation, consideration of other possible conditions, processes of care, and patient and family education and consent. However, withholding antibiotics while awaiting CT scan, laboratory studies, and admission to the hospital have all been shown to increase the time to antibiotic initiation for patients with suspected bacterial meningitis [7,97]. When bacterial meningitis is thought to be a likely diagnosis, antibiotics should be given just after an immediately performed LP, or if LP will be significantly delayed (such as after CT scan or in anticipation of prolonged transport time), antibiotics should be started soon after blood cultures are drawn [1,5,40,62,78]. Blood cultures are positive for the etiologic agent in approximately half to three quarters of cases of bacterial meningitis [4,6,40].

Prior to modern antibiotic therapy, pneumococcal meningitis had a mortality of 100%, and with the advent of effective antibiotics, the mortality rate has been reduced to 20% to 30% [6,98]. Thus, an infinite delay in antibiotic administration is clearly associated with worse outcomes. However, it is unclear exactly how time sensitive the initiation of antibiotics is in relation to patient outcomes. Existing data are limited by retrospective studies in which the duration of the meningitis infection (as opposed to a preceding viral or localized bacterial infection) is impossible to determine. A direct correlation between mortality and the duration of symptoms before beginning antibiotic therapy for patients with bacterial meningitis has not been consistently demonstrated [40]. A number of clinical features have been identified that independently predict worse patient outcome (eg, tachycardia, hypotension, seizures, altered mental status, CSF WBC count less than 1000) [4,6–8,10,99,100], and these potentially confounding factors need to be controlled in evaluating the association of antibiotic delay with outcomes [101,102]. Studies that have examined the relationship of patient outcome to the time to antibiotic initiation once bacterial meningitis was clinically suspected also have yielded inconsistent results [7,8,10,100], including three studies that attempted to control for other prognostic factors [7,8,100].

A retrospective cohort derivation and validation study of adverse outcomes in 269 adults with bacterial meningitis found no difference in time to antibiotics when controlling for patient prognostic stage, although it was noted that those patients who worsened to more advanced prognostic stages before antibiotics had worse outcomes than those who did not progress [8]. However, it is difficult to conclude that these findings were caused by antibiotic treatment delay, as rapid disease progression itself would be expected to predict worsened clinical outcomes regardless of antibiotic timing. Another retrospective investigation similarly found that delays of more than 6 hours from ED registration to antibiotic administration were independently associated with a greater risk of death [7]. These results are limited by the study design that evaluated 16 potential mortality-related factors among 123 patients with only 16 deaths. A prospective study of 156 adult ICU patients with pneumococcal meningitis with a mortality rate of 33% found that time to antibiotics after hospital presentation of longer than 3 hours was independently related to worse outcomes when controlling for illness severity [100]. The confidence in these findings is also limited, as multiple variables were evaluated and the 3-hour cut-off time was not prospectively defined.

The degree to which the time to initiate antibiotic therapy constitutes an inappropriate "delay" and what associated effect this may or may not have on patient outcomes raises frequent and contentious legal questions regarding negligence and causation. Unfortunately, if a bad outcome occurs after the diagnosis is confirmed, fair perspective is often lost for the difficult process of initial diagnosis. The diagnostic considerations involved in many of these cases are often challenging, and patients present with nonspecific findings that overlap with other diagnoses and may lack the constellation of typical features diagnostic of the uncommon diagnosis of meningitis. Although earlier treatment might logically be expected to increase the chance of an improved outcome, the available evidence is insufficient to assert that avoidance of a delay on the order of hours in any individual patient would prevent a bad outcome to a legal "more likely than not" standard. This issue is further confounded by the uncertainty of the time of onset of meningitis, the persistence of associated inflammatory reaction, and other potential factors that could affect prognosis.

Antiviral therapy for herpes simplex virus encephalitis

Viral encephalitis can be caused by a variety of pathogens that have no specific therapeutic options other than supportive care, such as adenoviruses, influenza A, and enteroviruses [103]. Some arbovirus encephalitis infections can be severe, such as those caused by West Nile virus or Eastern Equine Encephalitis. The most important treatable cause of encephalitis is HSV. HSV encephalitis leads to significant mortality if untreated (up to 70%), and even when immunocompetent patients are treated with appropriate antiviral therapy, there can be significant morbidity and mortality. Acyclovir has been demonstrated to be effective in significantly reducing mortality and is the empiric antiviral agent of choice for encephalitis [104–106]. Independent predictors of a poor outcome for patients with HSV encephalitis include Glasgow Coma Scale score of 6 or less, focal lesions found on CT scan of the head, increased patient age, and delays in initiating antiviral therapy longer than 4 days after onset [107–109]. Empiric therapy with acyclovir for encephalitis has been found to be started in only 29% of ED patients ultimately diagnosed with HSV [110]. Because altered mental status and focal neurologic abnormalities are key features of encephalitis, emergency care providers should consider empiric acyclovir in addition to antibiotic therapy in patients with these findings in whom the diagnosis of meningitis is also being considered.

Adjunctive corticosteroids for meningitis and encephalitis

Inflammation in the brain and spinal cord is poorly tolerated [111–113], and treatments to control the inflammatory responses to CNS infections may improve patient outcomes. Corticosteroids are recommended as an adjunctive therapy to reduce the inflammation associated with bacterial meningitis [114–117]. Children with bacterial meningitis caused by *H influenzae* type b have a reduced incidence of hearing loss with corticosteroid use, and protective effects are suggested when *S pneumoniae* is the pathogen [78]. A prospective, randomized, double-blind, multicenter, placebo-controlled trial of 301 adults with bacterial meningitis demonstrated that dexamethasone administered before or with the first dose of antibiotics and continued every 6 hours for 4 days led to significant improvement in patient outcomes [118]. Patients receiving dexamethasone had a reduced risk of an unfavorable outcome (relative risk [RR], 0.59; 95% CI, 0.37–0.94) and a reduced mortality (RR, 0.48; CI 0.24–0.96). Mortality in pneumococcal meningitis was reduced from 34% to 14% with steroid treatment [119].

A meta-analysis of 623 adult patients with bacterial meningitis demonstrated a decrease in mortality and neurologic morbidity associated with dexamethasone treatment [119]. The Cochrane Database review of randomized trials comparing corticosteroid therapy with placebo included 2750 adults and children and demonstrated an overall reduction in case fatality (overall RR, 0.83; RR for adults, 0.57), hearing loss (RR, 0.65), and long-term neurologic sequelae (RR, 0.67). Recommendations from this Cochrane review are to begin dexamethasone treatment before or at the same time as antibiotics in all adults and in children [120]. These recommendations emphasize that corticosteroids are to be administered just before or at the same time as antibiotic therapy, which is based on the totality of experimental and clinical studies, and emergency physicians should consider beginning corticosteroids at the time of empiric antibiotic administration [115,118,120–122].

Corticosteroids have also been recommended for the treatment of HSV encephalitis, in an effort to decrease the inflammation and thus reduce the morbidity and mortality of this disease. Although there are no large randomized controlled trials, recent studies using animal models of HSV encephalitis have demonstrated improved outcomes associated with corticosteroid treatment. Abnormalities found on brain MRI are reduced in mice with HSV-1 encephalitis when methylprednisolone is added to acyclovir treatment regimens [116]. Corticosteroids given 72 hours after HSV infection in mice led to neuroprotection and increased survival [123], although the mechanism underlying the clinical benefits is unclear. A small study in humans found that corticosteroid use in the acute phase of HSV encephalitis was a significant independent predictor of improved patient outcome and was the only identified potentially modifiable factor [109]. As patients with suspected HSV encephalitis are often also being treated empirically for possible bacterial meningitis, following current guidelines for corticosteroid treatment is recommended when encephalitis is considered, and current evidence suggests that this may also be beneficial should HSV encephalitis be later confirmed.

Patient disposition

Patients who are presumptively diagnosed with bacterial meningitis or encephalitis based on clinical findings, CSF results, and CNS imaging should be admitted to the hospital for monitoring, intravenous antimicrobial therapy, and adjunctive corticosteroids. However, some variability remains regarding patient disposition decisions in clinically well-appearing patients with mildly elevated levels of CSF WBCs but with other CSF findings suggestive of viral meningitis. The introduction of rapid CSF enteroviral PCR assays should allow outpatient management in many cases with a positive test result. Until this test is available, options for treatment of these patients pending the return of CSF culture results include hospital admission with continuation of empiric therapy or discharge with careful outpatient follow-up. Many such patients considered for discharge will have received initial dose(s) of empiric antibiotics, including ceftriaxone, which has a long duration of action. This further reduces the small risk of inadequately treated bacterial meningitis. Other factors to consider in patient disposition include patient reliability and social support systems, the availability of close follow-up care, and mechanisms for contacting patients if CSF culture results are positive. Careful return precautions should be provided to patients and family members for any signs of clinical worsening, and close outpatient follow-up should be arranged within 24 to 48 hours for re-evaluation to assess for any worsening or for other treatable causes of aseptic meningitis.

References

[1] Fitch MT, van de Beek D. Emergency diagnosis and treatment of adult meningitis. Lancet Infect Dis 2007;7(3):191–200.
[2] Schuchat A, Robinson K, Wenger JD, et al. Bacterial meningitis in the United States in 1995. Active Surveillance Team. N Engl J Med 1997;337(14):970–6.
[3] Durand ML, Calderwood SB, Weber DJ, et al. Acute bacterial meningitis in adults. A review of 493 episodes. N Engl J Med 1993;328(1):21–8.
[4] van de Beek D, de Gans J, Spanjaard L, et al. Clinical features and prognostic factors in adults with bacterial meningitis. N Engl J Med 2004;351(18):1849–59.
[5] van de Beek D, de Gans J, Tunkel AR, et al. Community-acquired bacterial meningitis in adults. N Engl J Med 2006;354(1):44–53.
[6] Weisfelt M, van de Beek D, Spanjaard L, et al. Clinical features, complications and outcome in adults with pneumococcal meningitis: a prospective case series. Lancet Neurol 2006;5(2):123–9.
[7] Proulx N, Frechette D, Toye B, et al. Delays in the administration of antibiotics are associated with mortality from adult acute bacterial meningitis. QJM 2005;98(4):291–8.
[8] Aronin SI, Peduzzi P, Quagliarello VJ. Community-acquired bacterial meningitis: risk stratification for adverse clinical outcome and effect of antibiotic timing. Ann Intern Med 1998;129(11):862–9.
[9] Hussein AS, Shafran SD. Acute bacterial meningitis in adults. A 12-year review. Medicine (Baltimore) 2000;79(6):360–8.

[10] Miner JR, Heegaard W, Mapes A, et al. Presentation, time to antibiotics, and mortality of patients with bacterial meningitis at an urban county medical center. J Emerg Med 2001; 21(4):387–92.

[11] Sigurdardottir B, Bjornsson OM, Jonsdottir KE, et al. Acute bacterial meningitis in adults. A 20-year overview. Arch Intern Med 1997;157(4):425–30.

[12] Schmutzhard E. Viral infections of the CNS with special emphasis on herpes simplex infections. J Neurol 2001;248(6):469–77.

[13] Ratzan KR. Viral meningitis. Med Clin North Am 1985;69(2):399–413.

[14] Baringer JR, Klassen T, Grumm F. Experimental herpes simplex virus encephalitis. Effect of corticosteroids and pyrimidine nucleoside. Arch Neurol 1976;33(6):442–6.

[15] Eisenstein LE, Calio AJ, Cunha BA. Herpes simplex (HSV-1) aseptic meningitis. Heart Lung 2004;33(3):196–7.

[16] Selbst SM, Friedman MJ, Singh SB. Epidemiology and etiology of malpractice lawsuits involving children in US emergency departments and urgent care centers. Pediatr Emerg Care 2005;21(3):165–9.

[17] Attia J, Hatala R, Cook DJ, et al. The rational clinical examination. Does this adult patient have acute meningitis? JAMA 1999;282(2):175–81.

[18] Green SM, Rothrock SG, Clem KJ, et al. Can seizures be the sole manifestation of meningitis in febrile children? Pediatrics 1993;92(4):527–34.

[19] Valmari P, Peltola H, Ruuskanen O, et al. Childhood bacterial meningitis: initial symptoms and signs related to age, and reasons for consulting a physician. Eur J Pediatr 1987;146(5): 515–8.

[20] Michos AG, Syriopoulou VP, Hadjichristodoulou C, et al. Aseptic meningitis in children: analysis of 506 cases. PLoS ONE 2007;2:e674.

[21] Oostenbrink R, Moons KG, Theunissen CC, et al. Signs of meningeal irritation at the emergency department: how often bacterial meningitis? Pediatr Emerg Care 2001;17(3): 161–4.

[22] Thomas KE, Hasbun R, Jekel J, et al. The diagnostic accuracy of Kernig's sign, Brudzinski's sign, and nuchal rigidity in adults with suspected meningitis. Clin Infect Dis 2002; 35(1):46–52.

[23] Uchihara T, Tsukagoshi H. Jolt accentuation of headache: the most sensitive sign of CSF pleocytosis. Headache 1991;31(3):167–71.

[24] Tyler KL. Herpes simplex virus infections of the central nervous system: encephalitis and meningitis, including Mollaret's. Herpes 2004;11(Suppl 2):57A–64A.

[25] Rennick G, Shann F, de Campo J. Cerebral herniation during bacterial meningitis in children. BMJ 1993;306(6883):953–5.

[26] Shetty AK, Desselle BC, Craver RD, et al. Fatal cerebral herniation after lumbar puncture in a patient with a normal computed tomography scan. Pediatrics 1999;103(6 Pt 1):1284–7.

[27] Horwitz SJ, Boxerbaum B, O'Bell J. Cerebral herniation in bacterial meningitis in childhood. Ann Neurol 1980;7(6):524–8.

[28] Oliver WJ, Shope TC, Kuhns LR. Fatal lumbar puncture: fact versus fiction–an approach to a clinical dilemma. Pediatrics 2003;112(3 Pt 1):e174–6.

[29] Masson CB. The dangers of diagnostic lumbar puncture in increased intracranial pressure due to brain tumor, with a review of 200 cases in which lumbar puncture was done. Research Nerv Ment Dis Proc 1927;8:422–34.

[30] Schaller WF. Propriety of lumbar puncture in intracranial hypertension. J Neurol Psychopathol 1933;14:116–23.

[31] Sencer W. The lumbar puncture in the presence of papilledema. J Mt Sinai Hosp N Y 1956; 23(6):808–15.

[32] Korein J, Cravioto H, Leicach M. Reevaluation of lumbar puncture; a study of 129 patients with papilledema or intracranial hypertension. Neurology 1959;9(4):290–7.

[33] Archer BD. Computed tomography before lumbar puncture in acute meningitis: a review of the risks and benefits. CMAJ 1993;148(6):961–5.

[34] Hasbun R, Abrahams J, Jekel J, et al. Computed tomography of the head before lumbar puncture in adults with suspected meningitis. N Engl J Med 2001;345(24):1727–33.

[35] Carpenter J, Stapleton S, Holliman R. Retrospective analysis of 49 cases of brain abscess and review of the literature. Eur J Clin Microbiol Infect Dis 2007;26(1):1–11.

[36] Thompson KA, Blessing WW, Wesselingh SL. Herpes simplex replication and dissemination is not increased by corticosteroid treatment in a rat model of focal Herpes encephalitis. J Neurovirol 2000;6(1):25–32.

[37] Cinque P, Cleator GM, Weber T, et al. The role of laboratory investigation in the diagnosis and management of patients with suspected herpes simplex encephalitis: a consensus report. The EU Concerted Action on Virus Meningitis and Encephalitis. J Neurol Neurosurg Psychiatr 1996;61(4):339–45.

[38] Carrol ED, Beadsworth MB, Jenkins N, et al. Clinical and diagnostic findings of an echovirus meningitis outbreak in the north west of England. Postgrad Med J 2006;82(963):60–4.

[39] Bernit E, de Lamballerie X, Zandotti C, et al. Prospective investigation of a large outbreak of meningitis due to echovirus 30 during summer 2000 in Marseilles, France. Medicine (Baltimore) 2004;83(4):245–53.

[40] Talan DA, Hoffman JR, Yoshikawa TT, et al. Role of empiric parenteral antibiotics prior to lumbar puncture in suspected bacterial meningitis: state of the art. Rev Infect Dis 1988;10(2):365–76.

[41] Zunt JR, Marra CM. Cerebrospinal fluid testing for the diagnosis of central nervous system infection. Neurol Clin 1999;17(4):675–89.

[42] Kanegaye JT, Soliemanzadeh P, Bradley JS. Lumbar puncture in pediatric bacterial meningitis: defining the time interval for recovery of cerebrospinal fluid pathogens after parenteral antibiotic pretreatment. Pediatrics 2001;108(5):1169–74.

[43] Pizon AF, Bonner MR, Wang HE, et al. Ten years of clinical experience with adult meningitis at an urban academic medical center. J Emerg Med 2006;30(4):367–70.

[44] Negrini B, Kelleher KJ, Wald ER. Cerebrospinal fluid findings in aseptic versus bacterial meningitis. Pediatrics 2000;105(2):316–9.

[45] Oostenbrink R, Moons KG, Twijnstra MJ, et al. Children with meningeal signs: predicting who needs empiric antibiotic treatment. Arch Pediatr Adolesc Med 2002;156(12):1189–94.

[46] Nigrovic LE, Kuppermann N, Malley R. Development and validation of a multivariable predictive model to distinguish bacterial from aseptic meningitis in children in the post-Haemophilus influenzae era. Pediatrics 2002;110(4):712–9.

[47] Freedman SB, Marrocco A, Pirie J, et al. Predictors of bacterial meningitis in the era after Haemophilus influenzae. Arch Pediatr Adolesc Med 2001;155(12):1301–6.

[48] Graham AK, Murdoch DR. Association between cerebrospinal fluid pleocytosis and enteroviral meningitis. J Clin Microbiol 2005;43(3):1491.

[49] Nigrovic LE, Kuppermann N, Macias CG, et al. Clinical prediction rule for identifying children with cerebrospinal fluid pleocytosis at very low risk of bacterial meningitis. JAMA 2007;297(1):52–60.

[50] Leblebicioglu H, Esen S, Bedir A, et al. The validity of Spanos' and Hoen's models for differential diagnosis of meningitis. Eur J Clin Microbiol Infect Dis 1996;15(3):252–4.

[51] Spanos A, Harrell FE Jr, Durack DT. Differential diagnosis of acute meningitis. An analysis of the predictive value of initial observations. JAMA 1989;262(19):2700–7.

[52] McKinney WP, Heudebert GR, Harper SA, et al. Validation of a clinical prediction rule for the differential diagnosis of acute meningitis. J Gen Intern Med 1994;9(1):8–12.

[53] Hoen B, Viel JF, Paquot C, et al. Multivariate approach to differential diagnosis of acute meningitis. Eur J Clin Microbiol Infect Dis 1995;14(4):267–74.

[54] Baty V, Viel JF, Schuhmacher H, et al. Prospective validation of a diagnosis model as an aid to therapeutic decision-making in acute meningitis. Eur J Clin Microbiol Infect Dis 2000;19(6):422–6.

[55] Jaeger F, Leroy J, Duchene F, et al. Validation of a diagnosis model for differentiating bacterial from viral meningitis in infants and children under 3.5 years of age. Eur J Clin Microbiol Infect Dis 2000;19(6):418–21.

[56] Oostenbrink R, Moons KG, Derksen-Lubsen AG, et al. A diagnostic decision rule for management of children with meningeal signs. Eur J Epidemiol 2004;19(2):109–16.

[57] Bonsu BK, Harper MB. Differentiating acute bacterial meningitis from acute viral meningitis among children with cerebrospinal fluid pleocytosis: a multivariable regression model. Pediatr Infect Dis J 2004;23(6):511–7.

[58] Ray P, Badarou-Acossi G, Viallon A, et al. Accuracy of the cerebrospinal fluid results to differentiate bacterial from non bacterial meningitis, in case of negative gram-stained smear. Am J Emerg Med 2007;25(2):179–84.

[59] Brivet FG, Ducuing S, Jacobs F, et al. Accuracy of clinical presentation for differentiating bacterial from viral meningitis in adults: a multivariate approach. Intensive Care Med 2005; 31(12):1654–60.

[60] Chavanet P, Schaller C, Levy C, et al. Performance of a predictive rule to distinguish bacterial and viral meningitis. J Infect 2007;54(4):328–36.

[61] Marton KI, Gean AD. The spinal tap: a new look at an old test. Ann Intern Med 1986; 104(6):840–8.

[62] Tunkel AR, Hartman BJ, Kaplan SL, et al. Practice guidelines for the management of bacterial meningitis. Clin Infect Dis 2004;39(9):1267–84.

[63] Maxson S, Lewno MJ, Schutze GE. Clinical usefulness of cerebrospinal fluid bacterial antigen studies. J Pediatr 1994;125(2):235–8.

[64] Hayden RT, Frenkel LD. More laboratory testing: greater cost but not necessarily better. Pediatr Infect Dis J 2000;19(4):290–2.

[65] Gerdes LU, Jorgensen PE, Nexo E, et al. C-reactive protein and bacterial meningitis: a meta-analysis. Scand J Clin Lab Invest 1998;58(5):383–93.

[66] Shimetani N, Shimetani K, Mori M. Levels of three inflammation markers, C-reactive protein, serum amyloid A protein and procalcitonin, in the serum and cerebrospinal fluid of patients with meningitis. Scand J Clin Lab Invest 2001;61(7):567–74.

[67] Sirijaichingkul S, Tiamkao S, Sawanyawisuth K, et al. C reactive protein for differentiating bacterial from aseptic meningitis in Thai patients. J Med Assoc Thai 2005;88(9): 1251–6.

[68] Knudsen TB, Larsen K, Kristiansen TB, et al. Diagnostic value of soluble CD163 serum levels in patients suspected of meningitis: comparison with CRP and procalcitonin. Scand J Infect Dis 2007;39(6):542–53.

[69] Uzzan B, Cohen R, Nicolas P, et al. Procalcitonin as a diagnostic test for sepsis in critically ill adults and after surgery or trauma: a systematic review and meta-analysis. Crit Care Med 2006;34(7):1996–2003.

[70] Gendrel D, Raymond J, Assicot M, et al. Measurement of procalcitonin levels in children with bacterial or viral meningitis. Clin Infect Dis 1997;24(6):1240–2.

[71] Viallon A, Zeni F, Lambert C, et al. High sensitivity and specificity of serum procalcitonin levels in adults with bacterial meningitis. Clin Infect Dis 1999;28(6):1313–6.

[72] Dubos F, Moulin F, Gajdos V, et al. Serum procalcitonin and other biologic markers to distinguish between bacterial and aseptic meningitis. J Pediatr 2006;149(1):72–6.

[73] Schwarz S, Bertram M, Schwab S, et al. Serum procalcitonin levels in bacterial and abacterial meningitis. Crit Care Med 2000;28(6):1828–32.

[74] Hoffmann O, Reuter U, Masuhr F, et al. Low sensitivity of serum procalcitonin in bacterial meningitis in adults. Scand J Infect Dis 2001;33(3):215–8.

[75] Kost CB, Rogers B, Oberste MS, et al. Multicenter beta trial of the GeneXpert enterovirus assay. J Clin Microbiol 2007;45(4):1081–6.

[76] Peltola H. Worldwide Haemophilus influenzae type b disease at the beginning of the 21st century: global analysis of the disease burden 25 years after the use of the polysaccharide vaccine and a decade after the advent of conjugates. Clin Microbiol Rev 2000;13(2):302–17.

[77] Albrich WC, Baughman W, Schmotzer B, et al. Changing characteristics of invasive pneumococcal disease in Metropolitan Atlanta, Georgia, after introduction of a 7-valent pneumococcal conjugate vaccine. Clin Infect Dis 2007;44(12):1569–76.

[78] Quagliarello VJ, Scheld WM. Treatment of bacterial meningitis. N Engl J Med 1997; 336(10):708–16.

[79] Gutierrez Rodriguez MA, Garcia Comas L, Rodero Garduno I, et al. Increase in viral meningitis cases reported in the Autonomous Region of Madrid, Spain, 2006. Euro Surveill 2006;11(11):E0611033.

[80] Lee BE, Davies HD. Aseptic meningitis. Curr Opin Infect Dis 2007;20(3):272–7.

[81] Kupila L, Vuorinen T, Vainionpaa R, et al. Etiology of aseptic meningitis and encephalitis in an adult population. Neurology 2006;66(1):75–80.

[82] Kardos K, McErlean M. Recurrent aseptic meningitis associated with herpes simplex virus type 2. Am J Emerg Med 2006;24(7):885–6.

[83] Tapiainen T, Prevots R, Izurieta HS, et al. Aseptic meningitis: Case definition and guidelines for collection, analysis and presentation of immunization safety data. Vaccine 2007;31(25):5793–802.

[84] Periard D, Mayor C, Aubert V, et al. Recurrent ibuprofen-induced aseptic meningitis: evidence against an antigen-specific immune response. Neurology 2006;67(3):539–40.

[85] Rodriguez SC, Olguin AM, Miralles CP, et al. Characteristics of meningitis caused by Ibuprofen: report of 2 cases with recurrent episodes and review of the literature. Medicine (Baltimore) 2006;85(4):214–20.

[86] Wambulwa C, Bwayo S, Laiyemo AO, et al. Trimethoprim-sulfamethoxazole-induced aseptic meningitis. J Natl Med Assoc 2005;97(12):1725–8.

[87] Ishida K, Uchihara T, Mizusawa H. Recurrent aseptic meningitis: a new CSF complication of Sjogren's syndrome. J Neurol 2007;254(6):806–7.

[88] Miller E, Andrews N, Stowe J, et al. Risks of convulsion and aseptic meningitis following measles-mumps-rubella vaccination in the United Kingdom. Am J Epidemiol 2007;165(6): 704–9.

[89] Whitley R. Diagnosis and treatment of herpes simplex encephalitis. Annu Rev Med 1981; 32:335–40.

[90] Aurelius E, Johansson B, Skoldenberg B, et al. Encephalitis in immunocompetent patients due to herpes simplex virus type 1 or 2 as determined by type-specific polymerase chain reaction and antibody assays of cerebrospinal fluid. J Med Virol 1993;39(3):179–86.

[91] Heyderman RS. Early management of suspected bacterial meningitis and meningococcal septicaemia in immunocompetent adults–second edition. J Infect 2005;50(5):373–4.

[92] Kearney BP, Aweeka FT. The penetration of anti-infectives into the central nervous system. Neurol Clin 1999;17(4):883–900.

[93] Karlowsky JA, Thornsberry C, Critchley IA, et al. Susceptibilities to levofloxacin in Streptococcus pneumoniae, Haemophilus influenzae, and Moraxella catarrhalis clinical isolates from children: results from 2000–2001 and 2001–2002 TRUST studies in the United States. Antimicrob Agents Chemother 2003;47(6):1790–7.

[94] Draghi DC, Sheehan DJ, Hogan P, et al. In vitro activity of linezolid against key gram-positive organisms isolated in the united states: results of the LEADER 2004 surveillance program. Antimicrob Agents Chemother 2005;49(12):5024–32.

[95] Talan DA, Zibulewsky J. Relationship of clinical presentation to time to antibiotics for the emergency department management of suspected bacterial meningitis. Ann Emerg Med 1993;22(11):1733–8.

[96] Bryan CS, Reynolds KL, Crout L. Promptness of antibiotic therapy in acute bacterial meningitis. Ann Emerg Med 1986;15(5):544–7.

[97] Talan DA, Guterman JJ, Overturf GD, et al. Analysis of emergency department management of suspected bacterial meningitis. Ann Emerg Med 1989;18(8):856–62.

[98] Swartz MN. Bacterial meningitis–a view of the past 90 years. N Engl J Med 2004;351(18): 1826–8.

[99] Weisfelt M, van de Beek D, de Gans J. Dexamethasone treatment in adults with pneumococcal meningitis: risk factors for death. Eur J Clin Microbiol Infect Dis 2006; 25(2):73–8.

[100] Auburtin M, Wolff M, Charpentier J, et al. Detrimental role of delayed antibiotic administration and penicillin-nonsusceptible strains in adult intensive care unit patients with pneumococcal meningitis: the PNEUMOREA prospective multicenter study*. Crit Care Med 2006;34(11):2758–65.

[101] Radetsky M. Duration of symptoms and outcome in bacterial meningitis: an analysis of causation and the implications of a delay in diagnosis. Pediatr Infect Dis J 1992;11(9): 694–8 [discussion: 698–701].

[102] Bonadio WA. Medical-legal considerations related to symptom duration and patient outcome after bacterial meningitis. Am J Emerg Med 1997;15(4):420–3.

[103] Kennedy PG. Viral encephalitis: causes, differential diagnosis, and management. J Neurol Neurosurg Psychiatr 2004;75(Suppl 1):i10–5.

[104] Whitley RJ, Alford CA, Hirsch MS, et al. Factors indicative of outcome in a comparative trial of acyclovir and vidarabine for biopsy-proven herpes simplex encephalitis. Infection 1987;15(Suppl 1):S3–8.

[105] Whitley RJ, Alford CA, Hirsch MS, et al. Vidarabine versus acyclovir therapy in herpes simplex encephalitis. N Engl J Med 1986;314(3):144–9.

[106] Skoldenberg B, Forsgren M, Alestig K, et al. Acyclovir versus vidarabine in herpes simplex encephalitis. Randomised multicentre study in consecutive Swedish patients. Lancet 1984; 2(8405):707–11.

[107] Morawetz RB, Whitley RJ, Murphy DM. Experience with brain biopsy for suspected herpes encephalitis: a review of forty consecutive cases. Neurosurgery 1983;12(6):654–7.

[108] Marton R, Gotlieb-Steimatsky T, Klein C, et al. Acute herpes simplex encephalitis: clinical assessment and prognostic data. Acta Neurol Scand 1996;93(2–3):149–55.

[109] Kamei S, Sekizawa T, Shiota H, et al. Evaluation of combination therapy using aciclovir and corticosteroid in adult patients with herpes simplex virus encephalitis. J Neurol Neurosurg Psychiatr 2005;76(11):1544–9.

[110] Benson PC, Swadron SP. Empiric acyclovir is infrequently initiated in the emergency department to patients ultimately diagnosed with encephalitis. Ann Emerg Med 2006;47(1): 100–5.

[111] Koedel U, Scheld WM, Pfister HW. Pathogenesis and pathophysiology of pneumococcal meningitis. Lancet Infect Dis 2002;2(12):721–36.

[112] Fitch MT, Doller C, Combs CK, et al. Cellular and molecular mechanisms of glial scarring and progressive cavitation: in vivo and in vitro analysis of inflammation-induced secondary injury after CNS trauma. J Neurosci 1999;19(19):8182–98.

[113] Fitch MT, Silver J. CNS injury, glial scars, and inflammation: Inhibitory extracellular matrices and regeneration failure. Exp Neurol; 2007 May 31 [Epub ahead of print].

[114] van de Beek D. Brain teasing effect of dexamethasone. Lancet Neurol 2007;6(3):203–4.

[115] van de Beek D, de Gans J. Dexamethasone in adults with community-acquired bacterial meninigitis. Drugs 2006;66(4):415–27.

[116] Meyding-Lamade UK, Oberlinner C, Rau PR, et al. Experimental herpes simplex virus encephalitis: a combination therapy of acyclovir and glucocorticoids reduces long-term magnetic resonance imaging abnormalities. J Neurovirol 2003;9(1):118–25.

[117] Jubelt B. Dexamethasone for the treatment of tuberculous meningitis in adolescents and adults. Curr Neurol Neurosci Rep 2006;6(6):451–2.

[118] de Gans J, van de Beek D. Dexamethasone in adults with bacterial meningitis. N Engl J Med 2002;347(20):1549–56.

[119] van de Beek D, de Gans J, McIntyre P, et al. Steroids in adults with acute bacterial meningitis: a systematic review. Lancet Infect Dis 2004;4(3):139–43.

[120] van de Beek D, de Gans J, McIntyre P, et al. Corticosteroids in acute bacterial meningitis. Cochrane Database Syst Rev 2007;1:CD004405.

[121] Begg N, Cartwright KA, Cohen J, et al. Consensus statement on diagnosis, investigation, treatment and prevention of acute bacterial meningitis in immunocompetent adults. British Infection Society Working Party. J Infect 1999;39(1):1–15.

[122] McIntyre PB, Berkey CS, King SM, et al. Dexamethasone as adjunctive therapy in bacterial meningitis. A meta-analysis of randomized clinical trials since 1988. JAMA 1997;278(11): 925–31.

[123] Sergerie Y, Boivin G, Gosselin D, et al. Delayed but not early glucocorticoid treatment protects the host during experimental herpes simplex virus encephalitis in mice. J Infect Dis 2007;195(6):817–25.

ELSEVIER
SAUNDERS

Infect Dis Clin N Am 22 (2008) 53–72

INFECTIOUS
DISEASE CLINICS
OF NORTH AMERICA

Diagnosis and Management of Pneumonia in the Emergency Department

Gregory J. Moran, MD, FACEP, FAAEM[a,b,c,*],
David A. Talan, MD, FACEP, FAAEM, FIDSA[a,b,c],
Fredrick M. Abrahamian, DO, FACEP[a,c]

[a]David Geffen School of Medicine at University of California Los Angeles,
Los Angeles, CA, USA
[b]Department of Medicine, Division of Infectious Diseases, Olive View-University of California
Los Angeles Medical Center, 14445 Olive View Drive, North Annex, Sylmar,
CA 91342–1438, USA
[c]Department of Emergency Medicine, Olive View-University of California Los Angeles
Medical Center, 14445 Olive View Drive, North Annex, Sylmar, CA 91342–1438, USA

Pneumonia remains a major cause of death in developed countries [1]. Patients with community-acquired pneumonia (CAP) are most often managed in an outpatient setting. The mortality rate in this patient population is low (<1%) in contrast to patients who require hospitalization, who have a mortality rate of approximately 15%. Because most patients with pneumonia are managed by emergency and primary care physicians, infectious disease specialists tend to see a population of patients with pneumonia that is skewed toward more complicated and severe infections. Emergency physicians may be less inclined than infectious diseases specialists to pursue aggressive diagnostic testing and cultures, except in patients who are seriously ill. Whereas in the past decisions regarding initial antibiotic therapy were deferred to admitting primary care and consulting physicians, quality standards currently reinforce timely initiation of antibiotics in the emergency department (ED). The practicality and ultimate consequences of arbitrary time standards are debated, however. Pneumonia management remains challenging because of several constantly changing factors,

* Corresponding author. Department of Emergency Medicine, Olive View-University of California, Los Angeles Medical Center, 14445 Olive View Drive, North Annex, Sylmar, CA 91342–1438.

E-mail address: gmoran@ucla.edu (G.J. Moran).

0891-5520/08/$ - see front matter © 2008 Elsevier Inc. All rights reserved.
doi:10.1016/j.idc.2007.10.003
id.theclinics.com

including an expanding spectrum of pathogens, changing antibiotic resistance patterns, the availability of newer antimicrobial agents, and increasing emphasis on cost effectiveness and outpatient management.

For patients with classic complaints of fever and productive cough, the clinical diagnosis of pneumonia is straightforward, especially when accompanied by pulmonary infiltrate on plain chest radiographs. More challenging, however, is identifying pneumonia in patients who present with atypical complaints (eg, abdominal pain). Once pneumonia is diagnosed, the priorities in the ED are to provide appropriate respiratory support, assess the severity of disease, initiate appropriate empiric antibiotic therapy based on the most likely pathogens, and make decisions regarding hospitalization and the need for isolation. Issues for which emergency physicians and infectious disease specialists may have different perspectives include the use of blood and sputum cultures, indications for hospital admission, appropriate level of care, and the breadth of antimicrobial spectrum for empiric therapy.

Diagnostic testing for pneumonia in the emergency department

Cough is a common presenting complaint; however, only a small fraction of patients who present with cough are diagnosed with pneumonia (4% in one large series) [2]. Patients with respiratory complaints should be screened with pulse oximetry at triage because hypoxia may not be otherwise clinically suspected, and its presence is an important diagnostic clue with therapeutic implications [3]. In most healthy older children and adults, the diagnosis of pneumonia can be reasonably excluded on the basis of history and physical examination, with suspected cases further evaluated by chest radiography. Absence of any abnormalities in vital signs or chest auscultation substantially reduces the likelihood of pneumonia. No single clinical finding, however, is highly reliable in establishing or excluding a diagnosis of pneumonia [4].

Chest radiography

Chest radiography is generally the most important test for establishing the diagnosis of pneumonia. Although it is clear that many chest radiographs are performed unnecessarily on patients with upper respiratory tract infections or bronchitis, it is difficult to identify a set of specific criteria to direct test ordering that is better than the clinical judgment of an experienced physician [5]. Routine chest radiography for all patients who present with cough is not necessary but may be reserved for patients without a history of asthma who have other suggestive findings (eg, fever, tachycardia, decreased oxygen saturation, or focal abnormality on lung examination) [6]. Among patients who are suspected of having pneumonia, these clinical findings have been prospectively validated and are better predictors of a radiographic infiltrate than physician judgment [7]. Patients with serious underlying disease or severe sepsis/septic shock in whom hospitalization is considered should have a chest radiograph performed. CT of the chest seems to be more sensitive than plain radiography for detecting the presence of pulmonary consolidation, although the natural history and clinical significance of CT-positive, plain radiograph-negative pneumonia are not clear [8]. CT may play a role in evaluating for other pulmonary diagnoses that may mimic pneumonia, such as pulmonary emboli, and may further delineate the nature of the pneumonia, such as in the case of necrotizing infection associated with community-associated methicillin-resistant *Staphylococcus aureus* (CA-MRSA).

Young, healthy adults with a presumptive diagnosis of pneumonia who are treated as outpatients may have chest radiography deferred unless there is a suspicion of immunocompromised status, tuberculosis (TB), or other unusual features of disease. Chest radiography should be performed subsequently if there is a poor initial response to treatment. Routine performance of chest radiography for patients with exacerbation of chronic bronchitis or chronic obstructive pulmonary disease is of low yield and may be limited to patients with other signs of infection or congestive failure [9]. Studies of infants with fever show that routine chest radiography is of low yield in the absence of other symptoms or signs of lower respiratory tract infection (eg, cough, rales, or elevated respiratory rate) [10,11]. One study found that leukocytosis was associated with occult pneumonia in children [12], but it is not clear whether identifying these cases has any clinical significance [13].

Rarely, patients with a clinical picture that strongly suggests pneumonia have a normal chest radiograph, and some are found to have an infiltrate noted within the next 24 to 48 hours. The absence of findings on a chest radiograph should not preclude the use of antimicrobial therapy in appropriate patients with a clinical diagnosis of pneumonia [14]. Whether the state of hydration can affect the radiographic appearance of pneumonia is unclear. Although severe dehydration theoretically could result in a diminished exudative response by decreasing blood volume and hydrostatic pressure, this finding has not been demonstrated in experimental models [15,16].

Laboratory studies

Laboratory studies are of limited use for establishing the diagnosis and specific cause of pneumonia. Although the finding of a white blood cell (WBC) count of more than $15,000/mm^3$ increases the probability of the patient having a pyogenic bacterial origin rather than a viral or atypical origin, this finding depends on the stage of the illness and is neither sensitive nor specific enough to aid decisions regarding therapy in an individual patient. A WBC count may be helpful if it reveals evidence of immunosuppression, such as neutropenia or lymphopenia, which may indicate immunosuppression from AIDS. Serum lactate dehydrogenase may be helpful in evaluating possible *Pneumocystis* pneumonia (PCP) in patients known or suspected to have HIV infection. Several rapid HIV tests are available that may be helpful in this situation [17]. Although CD4 counts usually cannot be obtained within the time frame of an ED visit, total lymphocyte count of less than $1000/mm^3$ predicts a higher likelihood of CD4 count less than $200/mm^3$ [18]. When suspicion exists for severe sepsis/septic shock, serum chemistry and coagulation studies may be helpful in evaluating patients for metabolic acidosis, renal and hepatic dysfunction, and disseminated intravascular coagulation. In the absence fluid-unresponsive hypotension, elevated arterial and central venous lactic acid levels also may indicate the need for early and aggressive hemodynamic resuscitation and broader empirical antibiotic therapy.

Patients with a pleural effusion should have a diagnostic thoracentesis performed with fluid sent for cell count, differential, pH (pH <7.2 predicts a need for chest tube), Gram stain, and culture. Although it is preferred to obtain pleural fluid specimen as early as possible, because of time constraints it is not always possible to perform diagnostic thoracentesis in every patient with pleural effusion in the ED. For most patients, thoracentesis can be deferred until after hospital admission. Patients in significant respiratory distress or with evidence of tension and mediastinal shift require emergent diagnostic and therapeutic thoracentesis, however. Assessment of respiratory function with pulse oximetry is important in the evaluation of patients with pneumonia. Because clinical assessment of oxygenation can be inaccurate [3], a pulse oximetry reading should be obtained in any patient suspected of having pneumonia in the ED—and ideally upon ED triage. Arterial blood gas measurement is usually unnecessary.

Identifying a specific etiologic agent

Many textbook discussions of pneumonia include clinical features that may predict a specific cause of pneumonia (eg, "currant jelly" sputum and bulging fissure on chest radiograph for *Klebsiella pneumoniae*, bullous myringitis for *Mycoplasma*). These findings have poor predictive value, however, and their presence or absence should not guide empiric therapy. Fortunately, recommended empiric regimens for CAP have activity against the most likely etiologies, so a specific etiologic diagnosis is usually unnecessary.

Pneumonia is often divided into two types: (1) "typical" pneumonia, which is caused by pyogenic bacteria, such as *Streptococcus pneumonia* or *Haemophilus influenzae,* and is characterized by productive cough with purulent sputum, high fever, and lobar consolidation, and (2) "atypical" pneumonia, which is caused by organisms such as *Mycoplasma pneumoniae* and *Chlamydophila pneumoniae* (formerly known as *Chlamydia pneumoniae*), and is characterized by a nonproductive cough with diffuse interstitial infiltrates. This differentiation is somewhat artificial; a clear differentiation between these two types of pneumonia on clinical grounds alone is impossible, and coinfection can occur. Factors studied prospectively and found not to be more frequent with atypical pneumonias than with pyogenic bacterial etiologies include gradual onset, viral prodrome, absence of rigors, nonproductive cough, lower degree of fever, absence of pleurisy, absence of consolidation, low leukocyte count, and an ill-defined infiltrate on chest radiograph [19].

Although it is impossible to determine with a high degree of certainty the specific cause of pneumonia without results of microbiologic or serologic tests, certain clinical features suggest a specific microbial cause. For example, a patient with known or suspected HIV and diffuse interstitial infiltrates should be evaluated for possible PCP. A severe, necrotizing pneumonia in the setting a previously healthy person with influenza should suggest CA-MRSA [20]. A patient with a history of intravenous drug use and plain chest radiograph with multiple focal infiltrates consistent with septic emboli should be suspected of having endocarditis, which is usually caused by S aureus (including MRSA). Geographic exposure to a current outbreak may lead to suspicion of infections such as avian influenza or severe acute respiratory syndrome.

Radiographic findings are poorly predictive of a particular infectious cause. For example, Mycoplasma pneumonia may present as a dense infiltrate, or pneumococcal pneumonia may present as a diffuse interstitial infiltrate. Immunocompromised patients are particularly prone to having atypical radiographic appearances. Findings such as apical pulmonary infiltrates, hilar adenopathy, and cavitation suggest TB, however, and should prompt initiation of appropriate isolation measures.

Sputum Gram stain and culture

Sputum Gram stain is often recommended as a means to determine the presence of a bacterial pathogen, allowing more specific antimicrobial therapy, but rarely results in a change in therapy or outcome. The routine use of sputum Gram stain as a basis for empiric therapy in the ED can be problematic for several reasons. Many patients are not able to provide an adequate sputum specimen. Induction of sputum without adequate isolation facilities can put patients and staff at risk if sputum is induced from persons with unrecognized TB. Correlation between identification of pneumococcus on Gram stain and sputum culture results is poor, even when commonly used criteria for an adequate sputum specimen (less than five squamous epithelial cells and >25 WBC/high power field) are applied. Gram stains are even less likely to demonstrate gram-negative pathogens, such as H influenzae, and should not be relied on to rule out a gram-negative cause.

Earlier recommendations regarding sputum analysis arose in the era of narrow spectrum antibiotics and may be less important in the era of broader spectrum agents that are given routinely for empirical treatment. Empirical antimicrobial agents are usually highly clinically effective if chosen based on clinical information without sputum analysis. With a high proportion of S pneumoniae strains resistant to penicillin, most physicians would not choose to treat a patient with penicillin even if a well-done sputum Gram stain revealed a predominance of gram-positive diplococci. The most recent Infectious Disease Society of America/American Thoracic Society (IDSA/ATS) consensus guidelines suggest that more aggressive diagnostic testing can be reserved for the more seriously ill patients. If sputum Gram stain and culture are considered, they should be reserved for the subset of patients with more serious illness (eg, admitted to the intensive care unit [ICU]), in whom the bacteriologic diagnosis is highly uncertain and for whom it is felt that the outcome may depend on optimal antimicrobial therapy. For example, in the ED, patients with pneumonia and respiratory failure who require intubation should have endotracheal suction specimens obtained.

Blood cultures

The need for routine blood cultures among patients admitted for pneumonia is also controversial [21,22]. Routine blood cultures for patients admitted with pneumonia have shown mixed results in terms of improved diagnostic accuracy or ability to guide therapy [23]. Most studies have revealed that the rates of false-positive culture results are similar to true-positive results, and false-positive culture results increase costs and prolong hospital stays [24,25]. In one prospective study of 760 patients with CAP, a change of antibiotic therapy based on blood cultures may have improved clinical outcome in only three cases (0.4%) [26]. Blood cultures should be obtained in seriously ill patients; if drawn, they should be obtained before the initiation of antibiotics (although antibiotics should not be delayed for this reason). When results are positive, blood cultures reflect the etiologic agent more accurately than sputum cultures but still only uncommonly lead to a rational change in antimicrobial therapy. Bacteremia occurs in approximately 25% to 30% of hospitalized pneumococcal pneumonia cases, but the diagnosis and therapy are usually well established before blood culture results are available.

It seems that blood cultures are useful for only a small fraction of admitted pneumonia patients, but it may be difficult to clearly identify who they are. Increasing reports of severe pneumonia caused by CA-MRSA illustrate the importance of pursuing the cause of pneumonia, at least in some cases [20,27,28]. It is reasonable to target patients with more severe illness for two reasons: (1) the incidence of bacteremia is higher [29] and (2) they have more to lose if empiric therapy is inappropriate.

The Joint Commission and the Centers for Medicare and Medicaid Services have removed routine blood cultures for all admitted patients as a quality measure, and the most recent edition of the IDSA/ATS guidelines for management of pneumonia does not recommend routine blood cultures for all admitted patients [1]. The Centers for Medicare and Medicaid Services still include a quality measure for obtaining blood cultures for patients admitted or transferred to the ICU within 24 hours of hospital arrival [30]. Unfortunately, it is often not possible to predict later transfer to ICU when a patient is admitted from the ED. Infectious disease consultants who see the minority of patients who deteriorate after initial treatment in the hospital may criticize the lack of blood cultures obtained on admission. Perspective from these occasional cases should not lead to a conclusion that all patients admitted with pneumonia need blood cultures. Blood cultures obtained from patients who do not show signs of serious infection at the time of ED evaluation are of lower yield and often give false-positive results (ie, contaminants). The follow-up of false-positive blood culture results can be costly and labor intensive and may lead to unnecessary use of agents such as vancomycin or linezolid when results are initially reported as gram-positive cocci in clusters.

The big decision: hospital or home?

Probably the single most important decision made in the ED is whether to admit a patient to the hospital or discharge home. Inpatient treatment of pneumonia is approximately 25 times more expensive per patient than outpatient treatment, and most patients are more comfortable in a home environment. There is tremendous variability in physician admission decisions for pneumonia. The more common tendency is overestimation of disease severity, which leads to hospitalization of patients at low risk for death or serious complications [31]. Although no firm guidelines exist regarding hospital admission, several well-recognized risk factors are associated with an increased risk of death or a complicated clinical course [32,33]. It is becoming more common practice for many hospitals and managed care systems to use some type of scoring system to assist with decisions regarding hospitalization for patients who have pneumonia.

One commonly used system is based on the Pneumonia Patient Outcomes Research Team study, a prospectively validated predictive rule for mortality among immunocompetent adults with CAP [34]. This model (also known as the pneumonia severity index [PSI]) suggests a two-step approach to assess risk. Patients in the lowest risk class who are recommended for outpatient management are younger than age 50, do not have significant comorbid conditions (eg, neoplasm, congestive heart failure, cerebrovascular disease, renal disease, liver disease), and do not have the following findings on physical examination: altered mental status, pulse 125 beats/min or more, respiratory rate 30 breaths/min or more, systolic blood pressure less than 90 mm Hg, or temperature less than 35°C or 40°C or more. Patients who do not fit the lowest risk category are classified into categories based on a scoring system that takes into account age, comorbid illness, physical examination findings, and laboratory abnormalities (Tables 1 and 2). Hospitalization is recommended for patients with a score more than 91 (class IV-V), and brief admission or observation may be considered for patients with a score of 71 to 90 (class III).

Table 1
Pneumonia severity index: scoring system for pneumonia mortality prediction

Patient characteristics	Points
Demographic factor	
Age	
Male	Years of age
Female	Years of age − 10
Nursing home resident	10
Comorbid illness	
Neoplastic disease	30
Liver disease	20
Congestive heart failure	10
Cerebrovascular disease	10
Renal disease	10
Physical examination finding	
Altered mental status	20
Respiratory rate >30	20
Systolic blood pressure <90 mm Hg	20
Temperature <35°C or >40°C	15
Pulse >125 beats/min	10
Laboratory or radiographic finding	
Arterial pH <7.35	30
Blood urea nitrogen >30 mg/dL	20
Sodium <130 mEq/L	20
Glucose >250 mg/dL	10
Hematocrit <30%	10
Arterial pO_2 <60 mm Hg	10
Pleural effusion	10

Adapted from Bartlett JG, Dowell SF, Mandell LA, et al. Practice guidelines for the management of community-acquired pneumonia in adults: Infectious Diseases Society of America. Clin Infect Dis 2000;31(2):347–82; with permission.

Although this method of assessing the likelihood of successful outpatient management is helpful in establishing general guidelines, it can be cumbersome to use, has not been modeled to predict acute life-threatening events, does not take into account dynamic evaluation over time, and has many important exceptions (eg, an otherwise low-risk patient with severe hypoxia would be discharged by strict interpretation of this rule). Additional discharge criteria could include improving and stable vital signs over a several-hour observation period, ability to take oral medications, an ambulatory pulse oximetry more than 90%, home support, and ability to follow-up. Good clinical judgment should supersede a strict interpretation of a scoring system. A study in which physicians were educated and provided the patient's risk score, however, revealed a significantly lower overall admission rate, cost savings, and similar quality-of-life scores compared with patients conventionally managed by their physicians [35]. Another study randomized patients in PSI class II-III to admission or discharge home and found that outcomes such as mortality and hospital readmission were similar, with higher patient satisfaction among outpatients [36]. EDs

Table 2
Risk classes and 30-day mortality rates for the pneumonia severity index

Risk class	Points	Mortality
I		0.1%
II	≤70	0.6%
III	71–90	0.9%
IV	91–130	9.3%
V	>130	27%

Data from Fine MJ, Auble TE, Yealy DM, et al. A prediction rule to identify low-risk patients with community-acquired pneumonia. N Engl J Med 1997;336(4):243–50.

that use higher intensity efforts to implement guidelines, including PSI, have lower admission rates for low-risk patients and higher compliance with antibiotic recommendations [37].

A similar tool that is easier to use is known as the CURB-65 rule [38]. This rule uses only five simple criteria to determine patients at lower risk for adverse events: Confusion, Uremia (blood urea nitrogen ≥20 mg/dL), Respiratory rate 30 breaths/min or more, Blood pressure less than 90 mm Hg systolic or 60 mm Hg or less diastolic, and age 65 or more. The risk of 30-day mortality increases with a greater number of these factors present: 0.7% with no factors, 9.2% with two factors, and 57% with five factors. It is recommended that patients with zero to one feature receive outpatient care, patients with two features be admitted, and ICU level care be considered for patients with three or more factors. No randomized trials of hospital admission strategies have directly compared the PSI to the CURB-65 score. In a comparison of scores in the same population of CAP patients, the PSI gave a slightly higher percentage of patients in the low-risk category, with a similar low mortality rate [39].

The disposition of HIV-infected patients with possible PCP is dictated by the likelihood of progression to severe disease and by the feasibility of close outpatient follow-up. Factors associated with decreased survival in patients who have AIDS and PCP include history of prior PCP, elevated respiratory rate, abnormal chest examination, WBC count more than $10,300/mm^3$, elevated lactate dehydrogenase, hypoxemia, hypoalbuminemia, and abnormal chest radiograph [40]. Patients without multiple poor prognostic factors or hypoxia may be discharged from the ED with close outpatient follow-up, ideally within 2 to 3 days.

The decision to hospitalize a patient with pneumonia is not necessarily a commitment to prolonged inpatient care. Twelve- to 24-hour ED or hospital ward observation may allow the early discharge of some patients. Other strategies sometimes used in the ED for patients with borderline indications for hospitalization include an initial parenteral dose of a longer half-life antibiotic, such as ceftriaxone, with a brief (eg, 2- to 6-hour) observation period. There are no evidence-based guidelines to identify which types of patients may be best managed with this strategy. Because these patients receive parenteral antibiotic therapy that would be equivalent to the antimicrobial component of inpatient care for the first day, it seems appropriate for intermediate-risk patients.

Level of care

In some cases it is obvious that a patient requires admission to an ICU, including patients who are intubated or require vasopressors for hemodynamic stabilization. It is more difficult to identify patients who do not require these interventions initially but may be at greater risk for deterioration and require a level of monitoring that may be beyond what is available on the typical hospital ward. Up to 45% of patients with CAP who ultimately require ICU admission are initially admitted to a non-ICU setting [41]. Transfer to the ICU for delayed onset of respiratory failure or septic shock is associated with increased mortality [42]. Defining "severe" pneumonia also has implications for empiric antimicrobial selection. Most studies of "severe" pneumonia have simply defined it as pneumonia in a patient admitted to the ICU. Objective criteria using the PSI (class V) and CURB-65 have been proposed but have not been prospectively validated for the ICU admission decision. When these criteria were retrospectively studied in a cohort of CAP patients, they did not perform better than actual physician decisions [43]. The 2007 IDSA/ATS guidelines include criteria for defining severe CAP that are based on ATS minor criteria and CURB variables (Table 3) [1]. They recommend that either of the two major criteria is an indication for ICU admission and that presence of at least three minor criteria would indicate a need for ICU admission. They also acknowledge that prospective validation of these criteria is needed.

Physicians may prefer to "err on the side of caution" and admit lower-acuity patients to a higher level of care rather than risk later ICU transfer from the hospital ward. It is important to recognize that this practice comes with a cost that may put other patients at higher risk for morbidity and mortality, however. Many ICUs in US hospitals are operating at capacity or near capacity, and seriously ill patients are spending more time boarding in EDs when no beds are available. ED overcrowding has adverse impacts that include ambulance diversions and longer transport times, longer waiting times for patients (some of whom have serious illness that cannot be recognized until they are evaluated by a physician), and lower overall quality of care [44]. Transfer of a deteriorating patient to the ICU from the hospital ward is not necessarily a failure. Some of the appropriate reasons for admitting patients to the hospital are to observe them and quickly move them to a higher level of care if necessary.

Isolation and infection control

Most patients with CAP do not need respiratory isolation. Patients who are suspected of having a cause of pneumonia that could pose a threat of

Table 3
Criteria for severe community-acquired pneumonia

Minor criteria[a]
Respiratory rate[b] $\geq$30 breaths/min
PaO_2/FiO_2 ratio[b] $\leq$250
Multilobar infiltrates
Confusion/disorientation
Uremia (BUN level, $\geq$20 mg/dL)
Leukopenia[c] (WBC count, <4000 cells/mm^3)
Thrombocytopenia (platelet count, <100,000 cells/mm^3)
Hypothermia (core temperature, <36°C)
Hypotension requiring aggressive fluid resuscitation
Major criteria
Invasive mechanical ventilation
Septic shock with the need for vasopressors

Abbreviations: BUN, blood urea nitrogen; PaO_2/FiO_2, arterial oxygen pressure/fraction of inspired oxygen.

[a] Other criteria to consider include hypoglycemia (in patients who do not have diabetes), acute alcoholism/alcoholic withdrawal, hyponatremia, unexplained metabolic acidosis or elevated lactate level, cirrhosis, and asplenia.

[b] A need for noninvasive ventilation can substitute for a respiratory rate >30 breaths/min or a PaO_2/FiO_2 ratio <250.

[c] As a result of infection alone.

Adapted from Mandell LA, Wunderink RG, Anzueto A, et al. Infectious Diseases Society of America/American Thoracic Society consensus guidelines on the management of community-acquired pneumonia in adults. Clin Infect Dis 2007;44(Suppl 2):S27–72; with permission.

transmission to other patients (eg, influenza, varicella, TB, plague) should be isolated. Isolation should be instituted as early as possible in the ED [45]. Patients who have neutropenia are generally placed in reverse isolation. The ED is a high-risk area for transmission of TB [46]. In many public hospitals, most patients who have pulmonary TB initially present through the ED [47]. Patients at high risk for TB, such as homeless persons, substance abusers, immigrants, and medically underserved low-income populations, frequently use the ED for health care [48]. Patients with TB risk factors often are cared for at busy public hospitals with long waiting times and crowded waiting rooms, which increases risk of health care transmission. Most US EDs do not have TB isolation facilities that comply with recommendations of the Centers for Disease Control and Prevention [49].

Patients suspected of possible pulmonary TB because of a history of TB exposure, suggestive symptoms (eg, persistent cough, weight loss, night sweats, hemoptysis), or belonging to a group at high risk for TB (eg, homelessness, intravenous drug use, alcoholism, HIV risk, immigration from high-risk area) should be placed immediately into respiratory isolation until active TB can be ruled out by further evaluation, including chest radiography [50]. Several published prediction models have attempted to assist clinicians with deciding which patients require TB isolation [51–53]. These models are limited by the small number of patients included with TB, however, and some are complex point-assignment models that are not easily applied in the busy ED setting. A systematic review of nine clinical prediction rules for isolating inpatients with suspected TB found that self-reported TB skin test results and upper lobe chest radiograph abnormalities demonstrated the strongest association with the diagnosis of TB [54].

HIV-infected patients who present with pneumonia ideally should be isolated until TB can be evaluated by sputum smears for acid-fast bacilli, particularly individuals with other risk factors for TB. Chest radiography cannot be relied on to exclude TB in patients who have AIDS because it often demonstrates diffuse infiltrates as opposed to characteristic cavitary lesions. Depending on individual risk assessment, other patients with noncavitary pulmonary infiltrates, such as inner-city homeless persons or intravenous drug users, may need to be isolated for possible TB. EDs that frequently care for patients at risk for TB should adopt triage protocols to rapidly identify these individuals and get masks and expedited chest radiographs before patients, visitors, or staff are unnecessarily exposed.

Empiric antimicrobial treatment of pneumonia in the emergency department

Timing of antimicrobial therapy

As with any seriously ill patient in the ED, initial attention should focus on ensuring adequate oxygenation, ventilation, and perfusion. Patients with underlying asthma or chronic obstructive pulmonary disease who present in respiratory distress may benefit from bronchodilator therapy and corticosteroids. Seriously ill patients who present with severe sepsis or septic shock require fluid resuscitation and vasopressors [55]. In the ED, empiric antimicrobial therapy for pneumonia is started before a definite microbiologic cause is established. For seriously ill patients who require hospital admission, antimicrobial therapy should be initiated as soon as possible once a reasonable suspicion of pneumonia exists because timely administration of antimicrobial agents has been shown to improve outcomes for hospitalized CAP patients [56].

The Centers for Medicare and Medicaid Services and the Joint Commission established administration of antibiotics within 4 hours of ED presentation for adults admitted to the hospital for CAP as a quality measure. This policy was largely based on a 2004 study that showed that administration of antimicrobial agents within 4 hours of hospital arrival was associated with lower mortality and reduced length of stay for Medicare patients over age 65 [57]. For various reasons, many facilities have had difficulty meeting this standard in a high proportion of patients. EDs in many US cities face critical overcrowding issues, and patients with pneumonia who do not appear seriously ill at triage may spend hours in the waiting room before evaluation. Because the "clock starts ticking" when the patient arrives at triage, the 4-hour time limit may pass by the time a patient is evaluated by a physician. The diagnosis of pneumonia is not always straightforward, and even minimal diagnostic testing in the ED may put a patient beyond the 4-hour window. Much like the problem of retrospective judgment, case reviews based on the final hospital diagnosis of pneumonia are biased toward overestimating therapeutic delays of patients who initially appear to have other conditions, such as congestive heart failure [58,59]. Some facilities have even resorted to a policy of giving antibiotics upon arrival for any patient with respiratory complaints that might be possibly caused by pneumonia. This strategy may improve compliance with the standard but obviously leads to many patients receiving unnecessary antibiotics [60,61].

The most recent IDSA/ATS CAP treatment guidelines state that the first dose should be given in the ED (preferably within 6–8 hours of arrival to the ED) but do not designate a specific time threshold [1]. Giving the first dose in the ED rather than on arrival to the hospital ward is associated with more rapid time to first dose of antibiotic and shorter length of hospital stay [62]. A rush to treatment without a diagnosis of CAP can result in inappropriate antibiotic use, however.

Choice of antimicrobial agents

The antibiotics chosen should provide coverage of the likely causes based on clinical, laboratory, radiologic, and epidemiologic information. Although it is not possible to predict a specific cause of pneumonia with a high degree of accuracy, it is possible to choose empiric therapy that covers the likely pathogens without being unnecessarily broad spectrum. For most older children and adults with CAP, it is appropriate to choose empiric regimens with activity against *S pneumoniae*, *H influenzae*, and atypical organisms such as *C pneumoniae* and *M pneumoniae*. Recommendations for empiric therapy for CAP in adults are summarized in Tables 4 and 5.

CA-MRSA has rapidly emerged as the most common pathogen isolated in community-acquired skin and soft-tissue infections [63] and is increasingly recognized as a cause of CAP. CA-MRSA pneumonia typically presents as a severe, rapidly progressing pneumonia with sepsis, often in children or healthy young adults [20]. Antimicrobial agents with consistent in vitro activity against CA-MRSA isolates include vancomycin, trimethoprim-sulfamethoxazole, daptomycin, tigecycline, and linezolid. Optimal therapy for MRSA is a subject of current debate in light of increasing minimum inhibitory concentrations for vancomycin [64,65]. Post hoc subgroup analysis of clinical trials for health care–associated pneumonia found that linezolid treatment in the subgroups found to have MRSA was associated with improved survival compared with vancomycin [66]. Prospective trials are ongoing to determine whether a difference truly exists. Daptomycin is inactivated by pulmonary surfactant, so it would not be appropriate for

Table 4
Community-acquired pneumonia in adults: inpatient antimicrobial treatment

Clinical setting	Antibiotic regimen	Comments
Community-acquired, nonimmunocompromised	Ceftriaxone, 1 g, every 24 h + azithromycin, 500 mg, every 24 h IV or orally	Could substitute cefotaxime, ampicillin-sulbactam, or ertapenem for ceftriaxone
	Respiratory fluoroquinolone (levofloxacin, 750 mg, IV every 24 h, or moxifloxacin, 400 mg, IV every 24 h)	Treats most common bacterial and atypical pathogens Active versus DRSP
Severe pneumonia (ICU)	Ceftriaxone, 1g IV every 24 h + levofloxacin, 750 mg, IV every 24 h + vancomycin, 1g, IV every 12 h	Can substitute cefotaxime, cefepime, ertapenem, or β-lactam/β-lactamase inhibitor for ceftriaxone Can substitute moxifloxacin for levofloxacin Can substitute linezolid for vancomycin
Severe pneumonia with neutropenia, bronchiectasis, or recent hospitalization (risk for *Pseudomonas*)	Cefepime, 2 g, IV every 12 h + ciprofloxacin, 400 mg, IV every 12 h + vancomycin, 1g, IV every 12 h	Can substitute other antipseudomonal β-lactam, such as piperacillin-tazobactam, imipenem, or meropenem for cefepime Can substitute aminoglycoside plus macrolide for ciprofloxacin
Presumed *Pneumocystis* pneumonia	Trimethoprim-sulfamethoxazole, 160/800 mg IV every 6 h	Add ceftriaxone to TMP/SMX, if severe, until PCP confirmed Alternatives for sulfa allergy include pentamidine + third-generation cephalosporin; clindamycin + primaquine; atovaquone + ceftriaxone

Doses are for 70-kg adult with normal renal and hepatic function.
Abbreviations: DRSP, drug-resistant *S pneumoniae;* IV, intravenously.

empiric therapy of pneumonia. Although it is not necessary to provide empiric coverage of MRSA for all pneumonia cases, it should be strongly considered for patients with severe pneumonia associated with sepsis, especially persons with concurrent influenza, contact with someone infected with MRSA, or radiographic evidence of necrotizing pneumonia.

Patients in nursing homes or other extended care facilities are often brought to the ED when they develop an acute problem, such as dyspnea or fever. Depending on their level of activity, comorbid conditions, history

Table 5
Community-acquired pneumonia in adults: outpatient treatment

Clinical setting	Antibiotic regimen	Comments
Previously healthy, no antimicrobials in last 3 months	Doxycycline, 100 mg orally, twice a day	Preferred for adolescent/ young adult when likelihood of mycoplasma is high; variable activity versus *S pneumoniae*
	Azithromycin	Treats common typical bacterial and atypical pathogens
		Variety of dosing regimens: 500 mg once followed by 250 mg daily for 4 days; 500 mg orally daily for 3 days; 2 g orally extended-release suspension once
		Can substitute clarithromycin
Comorbidities or antimicrobials in last 3 months	Levofloxacin, 750 mg orally, daily for 5 days	Can substitute moxifloxacin or gemifloxacin
		Treats common typical and atypical bacterial pathogens; active versus DRSP Use if recently received β-lactam or macrolide
	Cefpodoxime, 200 mg orally, twice a day + azithromycin, 500 mg orally, daily	Use if recently received fluoroquinolones
		Can substitute cefdinir, cefprozil, or amoxicillin/ clavulanate for cefpodoxime Variable activity against DRSP

Doses are for 70-kg adult with normal renal and hepatic function.
Abbreviation: DRSP, drug-resistant *S pneumoniae*.

of prior antibiotic use, and hospitalization, these patients are at increased risk for infection with resistant organisms such as *Pseudomonas aeruginosa, K pneumoniae* (including strains producing extended spectrum β-lactamases), *Acinetobacter* species, and hospital-associated strains of MRSA. Other risk factors for infection with multidrug-resistant pathogens include (1) hospitalization for 2 or more days in an acute care facility within 90 days of infection, (2) attending a hemodialysis clinic, and (3) receiving intravenous antibiotic therapy, chemotherapy, or wound care within 30 days of infection. Any patient with pneumonia that fulfills any of these historical features, including patients from a nursing home or long-term care facility, is designated as having health care–associated pneumonia, which is associated with a greater likelihood of resistant pathogens, such as *Pseudomonas* and MRSA. Mortality is also higher than with CAP [67]. It is appropriate to give broader spectrum empiric therapy to patients with health care–associated pneumonia, usually with a combination of antimicrobial agents to increase the chance that at least one antibiotic is active against the causative pathogen. Appropriate combinations include an antipseudomonal β-lactam agent, such as piperacillin/tazobactam, cefepime, imipenem or meropenem, combined with either an aminoglycoside or a fluoroquinolone and vancomycin or linezolid to cover for MRSA [68].

Studies of antiviral agents for influenza have generally focused on uncomplicated cases, but the impact of treatment on patients hospitalized with influenza or bacterial complications of influenza is less clear. It is reasonable to add antiviral treatment for pneumonia patients with positive antigen or culture-positive influenza or begin empiric treatment in patients with compatible clinical findings when influenza is in the community [1]. Neuraminidase inhibitors, such as oseltamivir, are a better choice than amantadine and rimantadine because they are active against influenza A and B and because many strains currently circulating in the United States are resistant to these older agents [69,70].

Patients who have HIV present an extra challenge because of possible risk for opportunistic pathogens. Because of the potential toxicity of sulfamethoxazole/trimethoprim (TMP/SMX), empiric treatment with this agent for well-appearing outpatients with a low probability of PCP is generally not recommended. An empiric trial of a macrolide may be indicated for treatment of mild CAP in a patient at low risk for PCP (eg, recent CD4 count $> 350/\text{mm}^3$). Any deterioration on outpatient oral antibiotics should prompt admission for a more extensive evaluation. Some emergency physicians initiate oral outpatient therapy with TMP/SMX or an alternate drug for patients with a high probability of PCP and favorable clinical parameters, but this should only be done if a patient can be followed closely for continued diagnostic evaluation and observation for toxicity. It is best done in consultation with the patient's continuing care physician.

It is common practice to initiate outpatient therapy in moderately ill patients for whom hospitalization might be considered, with administration of an initial parenteral dose of a long-acting antibiotic such as ceftriaxone (plus an initial dose of macrolide) and extended observation (ie, 12–24 hours) while administering supportive care such as hydration, antipyretics, and bronchodilators before discharge on an oral regimen. Certain patients also might be brought back to the ED for follow-up in 24 hours, either in person or by telephone. An outpatient regimen of an oral respiratory fluoroquinolone is another option that may be advantageous for moderately ill patients who are considered borderline for hospitalization. These agents have more reliable activity against drug-resistant *S pneumoniae* and good oral absorption that provides serum levels comparable to parenteral therapy [71].

Summary

Emergency physicians encounter a spectrum of pneumonia patients that is different than that encountered by infectious disease specialists. Most patients who have pneumonia and present to the ED can be safely discharged home on empiric oral antimicrobial agents with minimal diagnostic testing. Emergency physicians must be skilled at identifying patients who may require more extensive diagnostic testing, have severe sepsis/septic shock, are at risk for opportunistic infections such as PCP, and for whom empiric therapy should be expanded to cover less common organisms, such as CA-MRSA. Empiric antibiotics should be initiated in the ED, but using arbitrary time cutoffs for initiating antibiotics as a quality measure for patients ultimately diagnosed as having pneumonia is problematic. Decisions regarding hospital admission and level of care are central to emergency medicine practice and can be aided with prognostic models. It is also important to initiate infection control measures in the ED when appropriate.

References

[1] Mandell LA, Wunderink RG, Anzueto A, et al. Infectious Diseases Society of America/American Thoracic Society consensus guidelines on the management of community-acquired pneumonia in adults. Clin Infect Dis 2007;44(Suppl 2):S27–72.

[2] Metley JP, Stafford RS, Singer DE. National trends in the use of antibiotics by primary care physicians for adult patients with cough. Arch Intern Med 1998;158(16):1813–8.

[3] Mower WR, Sachs C, Nicklin EL, et al. Effect of routine emergency department triage pulse oximetry screening on medical management. Chest 1995;108(5):1297–302.

[4] Metlay JP, Kapoor WN, Fine MJ. Does this patient have community-acquired pneumonia? JAMA 1997;278(17):1440–5.

[5] Singal BM, Hedges JR, Radack KL. Decision rules and clinical prediction of pneumonia: evaluation of low yield criteria. Ann Emerg Med 1989;18(1):13–20.

[6] Heckerling PS, Tape TG, Wigton RS, et al. Clinical prediction rule for pulmonary infiltrates. Ann Intern Med 1990;113(9):664–70.

[7] Emerman CL, Dawson N, Speroff T, et al. Comparison of physician judgment and decision aids for ordering chest radiographs for pneumonia in outpatients. Ann Emerg Med 1991; 20(11):1215–9.

[8] Syrjala H, Broas M, Suramo I, et al. High-resolution computed tomography for the diagnosis of community-acquired pneumonia. Clin Infect Dis 1998;27(2):358–63.

[9] Sherman S, Skoney JA, Ravikrishnan KP. Routine chest radiographs in exacerbations of chronic obstructive pulmonary disease: diagnostic value. Arch Intern Med 1989;149(11):2493–6.

[10] Bramson RT, Meyer TL, Silbiger ML, et al. The futility of the chest radiograph in the febrile infant without respiratory symptoms. Pediatrics 1993;92(4):524–6.

[11] Baraff LJ. Management of fever without source in infants and children. Ann Emerg Med 2000;36(6):602–14.

[12] Bachur R, Perry H, Harper MB. Occult pneumonias: empiric chest radiographs in febrile children with leukocytosis. Ann Emerg Med 1999;33(2):166–73.

[13] Green SM, Rothrock SG. Evaluation styles for well-appearing febrile children: are you a "risk-minimizer" or a "test-minimizer"? Ann Emerg Med 1999;33(2):211–4.

[14] Melbye H, Berdal BP, Straume B, et al. Pneumonia: a clinical or radiographic diagnosis? Scand J Infect Dis 1992;24(5):647–55.

[15] Hall FM, Simon M. Occult pneumonia associated with dehydration: myth or reality? Am J Radiology 1987;148(5):853–4.

[16] Caldwell A, Glauser FL, Smith WR, et al. The effects of dehydration on the radiologic and pathologic appearance of experimental canine segmental pneumonia. Am Rev Respir Dis 1975;112(5):651–6.

[17] Centers for Disease COntrol and Prevention. General and laboratory considerations: rapid HIV tests currently available in the United States. Available at: http://www.cdc.gov/hiv/topics/testing/resources/factsheets/rt-lab.htm. Accessed October 1, 2007.

[18] Blatt SP, Lucey CR, Butzin CA, et al. Total lymphocyte count as a predictor of absolute CD4+ count and CD4+ percentage in HIV-infected persons. JAMA 1993;269(5):622–6.

[19] Fang GD, Fine M, Orloff J, et al. New and emerging etiologies for community-acquired pneumonia with implications for therapy: a prospective multicenter study of 359 cases. Medicine 1990;69(5):307–16.

[20] Centers for Disease Control and Prevention. Severe methicillin-resistant *Staphylococcus aureus* community-acquired pneumonia associated with influenza: Louisiana and Georgia, December 2006–January 2007. MMWR Morb Mortal Wkly Rep 2007;56(14):325–9.

[21] Moran GJ, Abrahamian FM. Blood cultures for pneumonia: can we hit the target without a shotgun? Ann Emerg Med 2005;46(5):407–8.

[22] Walls RM, Resnick J. The Joint Commission on Accreditation of Healthcare Organizations and Center for Medicare and Medicaid Services community-acquired pneumonia initiative: what went wrong? Ann Emerg Med 2005;46(5):409–11.

[23] Kennedy M, Bates DW, Wright SB, et al. Do emergency department blood cultures change practice in patients with pneumonia? Ann Emerg Med 2005;46(5):393–400.

[24] Chalasani NP, Valdecanas MA, Gopal AK, et al. Clinical utility of blood cultures in adult patients with community-acquired pneumonia without defined underlying risks. Chest 1995;108(4):932–6.

[25] Corbo J, Friedman B, Bijur P, et al. Limited usefulness of initial blood cultures in community acquired pneumonia. Emerg Med J 2004;21(4):446–8.

[26] Campbell SG, Marrie TJ, Anstey R, et al. The contribution of blood cultures to the clinical management of adult patients admitted to the hospital with community-acquired pneumonia: a prospective observational study. Chest 2003;123(4):1142–50.

[27] Frazee BW, Salz TO, Lambert L, et al. Fatal community-associated methicillin-resistant *Staphylococcus aureus* pneumonia in an immunocompetent young adult. Ann Emerg Med 2005;46(5):401–4.

[28] Hageman JC, Uyeki TM, Francis JS, et al. Severe community-acquired pneumonia due to *Staphylococcus aureus*, 2003–04 influenza season. Emerg Infect Dis 2006;12(6):894–9.

[29] Mandell LA, Marrie TJ, Grossman RF, et al. Canadian guidelines for the initial management of community-acquired pneumonia: an evidence-based update by the Canadian Infectious Diseases Society and the Canadian Thoracic Society. The Canadian Community-Acquired Pneumonia Working Group. Clin Infect Dis 2000;31(2):383–421.

[30] Agency for Healthcare Research and Quality. National quality measures clearinghouse: pneumonia. Available at: http://www.qualitymeasures.ahrq.gov/summary/summary.aspx?doc_id=9499. Accessed October 1, 2007.

[31] McMahon LF Jr, Wolfe RA, Tedeschi PJ. Variation in hospital admission among small areas: a comparison of Maine and Michigan. Med Care 1989;27(6):623–31.

[32] Fine MJ, Smith DN, Singer DE. Hospitalization decision in patients with community-acquired pneumonia: a prospective cohort study. Am J Med 1990;89(6):713–21.

[33] Black ER, Mushlin AI, Griner PF, et al. Predicting the need for hospitalization of ambulatory patients with pneumonia. J Gen Intern Med 1991;6(5):394–400.

[34] Fine MJ, Auble TE, Yealy DM, et al. A prediction rule to identify low-risk patients with community-acquired pneumonia. N Engl J Med 1997;336(4):243–50.

[35] Marrie TJ, Lau CY, Wheeler SL, et al. A controlled trial of a critical pathway for treatment of community-acquired pneumonia. JAMA 2000;283(6):749–55.

[36] Carratala J, Fernandez-Sabe N, Ortega L, et al. Outpatient care compared with hospitalization for community-acquired pneumonia: a randomized trial in low-risk patients. Ann Intern Med 2005;142(3):165–72.

[37] Yealy DM, Auble TE, Stone RA, et al. Effect of increasing the intensity of implementing pneumonia guidelines: a randomized, controlled trial. Ann Intern Med 2005;143(12):881–94.

[38] Lim WS, van der Eerden MM, Liang R, et al. Defining community-acquired pneumonia severity on presentation to hospital: an international derivation and validation study. Thorax 2003;58(5):377–82.

[39] Aujesky D, Auble TE, Yealy DM, et al. Prospective comparison of three validated prediction rules for prognosis in community-acquired pneumonia. Am J Med 2005;118(4):384–92.

[40] Masur H. Prevention and treatment of Pneumocystis pneumonia. N Engl J Med 1992; 327(26):1853–60.

[41] Ewig S, de Roux A, Bauer T, et al. Validation of predictive rules and indices of severity for community-acquired pneumonia. Thorax 2004;59(5):421–7.

[42] Leroy O, Santre C, Beuscart C, et al. A five-year study of severe community-acquired pneumonia with emphasis on prognosis in patients admitted to an intensive care unit. Intensive Care Med 1995;21(1):24–31.

[43] Angus DC, Marrie TJ, Obrosky DS, et al. Severe community-acquired pneumonia: use of intensive care services and evaluation of American and British Thoracic Society Diagnostic criteria. Am J Respir Crit Care Med 2002;166(5):717–23.

[44] Committee on the Future of Emergency Care in the United States Health System. Hospital-based emergency care: at the breaking point. Washington, DC: National Academies Press; 2006.

[45] Rothman RE, Irvin CB, Moran GJ, et al. Respiratory hygiene in the emergency department. Ann Emerg Med 2006;48(5):570–82.

[46] Sokolove PE, Mackey D, Wiles J, et al. Exposure of emergency department personnel to tuberculosis: PPD testing during an epidemic in the community. Ann Emerg Med 1994;24(3): 418–21.

[47] Moran GJ, McCabe F, Morgan MT, et al. Delayed recognition and infection control for tuberculosis patients in the emergency department. Ann Emerg Med 1995;26(3):290–5.

[48] Baker DW, Stevens CD, Brook RH. Regular source of ambulatory care and medical care utilization by patients presenting to a public hospital emergency department. JAMA 1994; 271(24):1909–12.

[49] Moran GJ, Fuchs MA, Jarvis WR, et al. Tuberculosis infection-control practices in United States emergency departments. Ann Emerg Med 1995;26(3):283–9.

[50] Centers for Disease Control and Prevention. Guidelines for preventing the transmission of *Mycobacterium tuberculosis* in health-care facilities, 1994. MMWR Recomm Rep 1994; 43(RR-13):1–132.

[51] El-Solh A, Mylotte J, Sherif S, et al. Validity of a decision tree for predicting active pulmonary tuberculosis. Am J Respir Crit Care Med 1997;155(5):1711–6.

[52] Tattevin P, Casalino E, Fleury L, et al. The validity of medical history, classic symptoms, and chest radiographs in predicting pulmonary tuberculosis. Chest 1999;115(5):1248–53.

[53] Wisnivesky JP, Henschke C, Balentine J, et al. Prospective validation of a prediction model for isolating inpatients with suspected pulmonary tuberculosis. Arch Intern Med 2005; 165(4):453–7.

[54] Wisnivesky JP, Serebrisky D, Moor C, et al. Validity of clinical prediction rules for isolating inpatients with suspected tuberculosis: a systematic review. J Gen Intern Med 2005;20(10): 947–52.

[55] Nguyen HB, Rivers EP, Abrahamian FM, et al. Severe sepsis and septic shock: review of the literature and emergency department management guidelines. Ann Emerg Med 2006;48(1): 28–54.

[56] Meehan TP, Fine MJ, Krumholz HM, et al. Quality of care, process, and outcomes in elderly patients with pneumonia. JAMA 1997;278(23):2080–4.

[57] Houck PM, Bratzler DW, Nsa W, et al. Timing of antibiotic administration and outcomes for Medicare patients hospitalized with community-acquired pneumonia. Arch Intern Med 2004;164(6):637–44.

[58] Pines JM, Morton MF, Datner EM, et al. Systematic delays in antibiotic administration in the emergency department for adult patients admitted with pneumonia. Acad Emerg Med 2006;13(9):939–45.

[59] Fee C, Weber EJ. Identification of 90% of patients ultimately diagnosed with community-acquired pneumonia within four hours of emergency department arrival may not be feasible. Ann Emerg Med 2007;49(5):553–9.

[60] Pines JM, Hollander JE, Lee H, et al. Emergency department operational changes in response to pay-for-performance and antibiotic timing in pneumonia. Acad Emerg Med 2007;14(6):545–8.

[61] Kelen GD, Rothman RE. Community pneumonia practice standard mandates: can't see the forest for the trees. Acad Emerg Med 2006;13(9):986–8.

[62] Battleman DS, Callahan M, Thaler HT. Rapid antibiotic delivery and appropriate antibiotic selection reduce length of hospital stay of patients with community-acquired pneumonia. Arch Intern Med 2002;162(6):682–8.

[63] Moran GJ, Krishnadasan A, Gorwitz RJ, et al, for The EMERGEncy ID NET Study Group. Methicillin-resistant S. aureus infections among patients in the emergency department. N Engl J Med 2006;355(7):666–74.

[64] Mohr JF, Murray BE. Point: vancomycin is not obsolete for the treatment of infection caused by methicillin-resistant Staphylococcus aureus. Clin Infect Dis 2007;44(12):1536–42.

[65] Deresinski S. Counterpoint: vancomycin and Staphylococcus aureus. An antibiotic enters obsolescence. Clin Infect Dis 2007;44(12):1543–8.

[66] Wunderink RG, Rello J, Cammarate SK, et al. Linezolid vs. vancomycin: analysis of two double-blind studies of patients with methicillin-resistant Staphylococcus aureus nosocomial pneumonia. Chest 2003;124(5):1789–97.

[67] Kollef MH, Shorr A, Tabak YP, et al. Epidemiology and outcomes of health-care-associated pneumonia: results from a large US database of culture-positive pneumonia. Chest 2005;128(6):3854–62.

[68] American Thoracic Society. Guidelines for the management of adults with hospital-acquired, ventilator-associated, and healthcare-associated pneumonia. Am J Respir Crit Care Med 2005;171(4):388–416.

[69] Gubareva LV, Kaiser L, Hayden FG. Influenza virus neuraminidase inhibitors. Lancet 2000;355(9206):827–35.

[70] Centers for Disease Control and Prevention. High levels of adamantane resistance among influenza A (H3N2) viruses and interim guidelines for use of antiviral agents: United States, 2005–06 influenza season. MMWR Morb Mortal Wkly Rep 2006;55(02):44–6.

[71] Moran GJ. Approaches to treatment of community-acquired pneumonia in the emergency department and the appropriate role of fluoroquinolones. J Emerg Med 2006;30(4):377–87.

ELSEVIER
SAUNDERS

INFECTIOUS
DISEASE CLINICS
OF NORTH AMERICA

Infect Dis Clin N Am 22 (2008) 73–87

Urinary Tract Infections in the Emergency Department

Fredrick M. Abrahamian, DO, FACEP[a,b,*],
Gregory J. Moran, MD, FACEP, FAAEM[a,b,c],
David A. Talan, MD, FACEP, FAAEM, FIDSA[a,b,c]

[a]David Geffen School of Medicine at University of California Los Angeles,
Los Angeles, CA, USA
[b]Department of Emergency Medicine, Olive View-University of California Los Angeles
Medical Center, Sylmar, CA, USA
[c]Department of Medicine, Division of Infectious Diseases, Olive View-University of California
Los Angeles Medical Center, Sylmar, CA, USA

Urinary tract infection (UTI) is a commonly encountered clinical condition in the emergency department (ED). The spectrum of disease severity as seen by emergency physicians is wide and can range from uncomplicated cystitis to pyelonephritis and fulminant urosepsis syndrome. Infectious disease (ID) specialists, on the other hand, are most often consulted on patients with complicated UTIs and those who are admitted to the hospital with more severe illness. This article is written from the perspective of the evaluation and initial management of UTIs in the ED. The pitfalls and clinical dilemmas pertinent to emergency physicians that are not often encountered by ID specialists are highlighted.

Classification

Various classification schemes have been used to subdivide UTIs in adults: upper tract versus lower tract, complicated versus uncomplicated, symptomatic versus asymptomatic. However, in practice, especially in the ED, it is often difficult to make clinical decisions based solely on one classification scheme on account of the considerable overlap among them. In the ED, symptomatic UTIs in adults are often categorized as an uncomplicated UTI (cystitis or

* Corresponding author. Department of Emergency Medicine, Olive View-University of California Los Angeles Medical Center, 14445 Olive View Drive, North Annex, Sylmar, CA 91342–1438.
E-mail address: fmasjc@ucla.edu (F.M. Abrahamian).

0891-5520/08/$ - see front matter © 2008 Elsevier Inc. All rights reserved.
doi:10.1016/j.idc.2007.10.002
id.theclinics.com

pyelonephritis) occurring in a woman versus a complicated UTI occurring in a woman or man. Uncomplicated infections are generally considered to occur in healthy, premenopausal, nonpregnant females without comorbidities, structural defects in urinary anatomy, or renal function abnormalities.

Complicated infections are defined for patient populations such as those at extremes of age, male gender, the presence of anatomic or functional abnormality (eg, obstruction, neurogenic bladder), concurrent urolithiasis, presence of foreign body (eg, catheter), immunosuppressed state (eg, diabetes, malignancy), pregnancy, history of recent instrumentation, or the presence of an unusual or resistant organism. Recent antibiotic use, multiple recurrent infections, age of 65 years or older, the presence of urinary tract abnormalities, and long-lasting symptoms increase the probability of resistant organisms causing the infection [1–5]. UTIs in men are generally considered complicated as most of them occur in association with other conditions such as sexually transmitted diseases (STDs), urinary retention, prostatitis, urologic anatomic abnormalities, or urinary tract instrumentation.

Microbiology

The etiology of UTI depends on several factors: patient's age, underlying medical conditions (eg, diabetes, spinal cord injury), type of infection (complicated versus uncomplicated), and history of antibiotic use or hospitalization in the preceding 3 months. In the majority of patients with uncomplicated cystitis and pyelonephritis, the infection is monobacterial with *Escherichia coli*; *Staphylococcus saprophyticus* can be encountered in approximately 10% of young women with acute uncomplicated cystitis. Compared with uncomplicated infections, the proportion of cases due to *Pseudomonas aeruginosa*, or *Enterococcus*, *Klebsiella*, *Proteus*, and *Enterobacter* sp is much greater in complicated infections [6]. Polymicrobial infections are also more frequently encountered in complicated infections.

Clinical presentation

Acute cystitis is a common infection, especially in young adult women. The clinical presentation can be variable with one or more symptoms of UTI such as dysuria, urinary frequency, hematuria, urgency, and suprapubic discomfort. In an evidence-based review, the probability of a UTI in a patient presenting with one or more symptoms of UTI (eg, dysuria, frequency, hematuria) was approximately 50% (positive likelihood ratio [LR+] of 19). The probability increased to 96% (LR+ = 24.6) if the patient presented with the triad of dysuria, frequency, and no vaginal symptoms [7].

A pitfall to relying solely on the symptoms of dysuria, urinary frequency, and urgency is that they are not specific for UTI and can be observed with STDs, vaginitis, and non-infectious conditions (eg, chemical, allergic, traumatic events). In addition, clinical signs and symptoms do not consistently or accurately differentiate UTI from early STDs, and high rates of concurrent disease are common especially in the young urban population [8–10]. However, absence of dysuria and back pain, in combination with a history of vaginal discharge and irritation and vaginal discharge on pelvic examination, decreases the probability of UTI [7].

Acute pyelonephritis is a clinical syndrome characterized by fever, chills, and flank pain or tenderness—usually accompanied by symptoms of a lower UTI (eg, frequency, urgency, dysuria)—and is subsequently found to have bacteriuria. Owing to the severity of symptoms, patients with pyelonephritis are more likely to seek medical care and visit EDs than patients with acute cystitis.

Unusual presentations of pyelonephritis are common, and some patients may lack the classic symptoms of UTI and present with only flank pain and costovertebral angle tenderness. A few patients may describe the pain associated with pyelonephritis in atypical locations such as the epigastric region, or right or left upper abdominal quadrants. Fever is commonly present, and its absence should heighten suspicion for the presence of other clinical conditions. In a retrospective cohort study of women 15 years of age or older admitted to the hospital with the diagnosis of pyelonephritis, those patients lacking fever (temperature less than 37.8°C) were more often found to have other diagnoses such as cholecystitis, pelvic inflammatory disease, and diverticulitis [11].

The presentation of pyelonephritis can be particularly challenging in the elderly. These patients may be afebrile or have only a low-grade temperature on presentation. They may not be able to verbalize their symptoms (eg, patients with dementia or stroke) and may present with altered mental status, lethargy, or complaints of abdominal pain or generalized weakness.

The absence of commonly observed symptoms of acute pyelonephritis does not exclude the existence of infection. "Subclinical" pyelonephritis can be present in patients with characteristic symptoms of acute cystitis [12,13]. Patients who are at higher risk for subclinical pyelonephritis include those with complicating features such as history of recurrent UTIs, patients with persistent long-standing symptoms (ie, greater than 7 days), those who have failed short-course UTI therapy, male gender, patients with diabetes, pregnancy, and immunosuppression. In clinical practice, the diagnosis of subclinical pyelonephritis is most often retrospective and is suspected in patients who failed initial therapy for acute cystitis.

Laboratory evaluation

In most adults presenting to the ED, a urine specimen is collected through the midstream-voiding technique. In a prospective study of 105 women with UTI symptoms, there were no statistically significant differences in urinalysis findings or the rate of positive urine cultures when urine was obtained through a midstream clean-catch or in-and-out catheterization

[14]. Catheterization becomes necessary if the patient is unable to void spontaneously. Other situations that necessitate catheterization in the ED include patient too ill or immobilized, unable to follow instructions, extreme obesity, or if the patient has a concomitant condition that may result in the contamination of urine (eg, vaginal discharge or bleeding).

The key laboratory test relied on to diagnose UTI in the ED is through microscopic examination of the urine. The presence of pyuria on urinalysis has a sensitivity of 95% and a specificity of 71% for UTI [15]. The absence of pyuria should make one consider other diagnoses.

Some patients with classic symptoms of UTI encountered in the ED occasionally have a negative urinalysis. A negative urinalysis or urine dipstick test does not completely exclude the presence of UTI in patients with one or more symptoms of UTI [7,16,17], especially those who have had past history of documented UTI (high pretest probability). These patients pose a diagnostic dilemma and, as a result, therapeutic decisions become challenging. Various factors can cause a negative urinalysis in such patients and include low-level pyuria or bacteriuria and recent antibiotic exposure. Contrary to common belief, high fluid intake (ie, dilute urine) has not been shown to result in low-count bacteriuria (ie, $>10^2-10^4$ colony-forming units [CFU]/mL) [18]. In patients with classic symptoms of UTI and a negative urinalysis, a common clinical practice—although not unique to the ED—is to obtain a urine culture, initiate antimicrobial therapy for UTI, and exclude other potential causes for the symptoms (eg, STDs). In a prospective, double-blind, randomized, placebo-controlled trial of 59 women 16 to 50 years of age and presenting with complaints of dysuria and frequency and a negative urine dipstick test for leukocytes and nitrites, 3 days of antimicrobial therapy significantly reduced dysuria. At the completion of therapy, 76% of patients who received antibiotics reported resolution of dysuria as compared with 26% of women in the placebo group ($P = .0005$). At day 7, 90% of the treated women reported resolution of dysuria as compared with 59% of women in the placebo group ($P = .02$) (number needed to treat = 4) [19].

Although urine culture is the traditional reference standard for confirming the diagnosis of UTI, owing to the delay in its turnaround time it provides no immediate diagnostic utility for emergency physicians. Pretreatment urine cultures are often not performed in patients who present with signs and symptoms compatible with acute uncomplicated cystitis. In these patients, the routine performance of urine cultures has not been shown to be cost effective or predictive of the therapeutic outcome [20,21]. However, these studies were conducted when resistance to standard UTI therapies such as trimethoprim-sulfamethoxazole (TMP/SMX) and fluoroquinolones was not so prevalent. In the current era of increasing resistance, especially as resistance has been shown to translate into clinical and microbiologic failure [22], there may be justification for routinely culturing patients with uncomplicated infections. Certainly, this is an area of debate and further studies are warranted. In contrast, urine culture and susceptibility tests are of diagnostic value, and are commonly performed in patients with pyelonephritis and those with complicated infections. Cultures are also warranted for patients whose symptoms either do not resolve or recur soon after the completion of therapy.

The routine performance of blood cultures is not recommended in patients with acute uncomplicated cystitis, owing to the localized nature of the infection and rarity of bacteremia. Various studies have investigated the utility of blood cultures in patients with pyelonephritis [23–29]. Overall, blood cultures have been shown to have limited clinical value in premenopausal women with acute uncomplicated pyelonephritis. In a prospective study of 583 women with acute uncomplicated pyelonephritis, blood cultures were seldom different from urine cultures, and no single case required a change in antimicrobial therapy based on blood culture results [23]. Similar results have also been recognized in pregnant patients with pyelonephritis [24,25]. Discordant results are more commonly observed in postmenopausal women [23]. Contamination of blood culture by skin flora is a common cause of the discrepancies between blood and urine cultures. The routine performance of blood cultures is costly and time consuming. False-positive results further complicate management decisions and introduce confusion. On the basis of the available evidence, it is best to reserve blood cultures for postmenopausal women and those with complicated infections [30].

Imaging

Other diagnostic tests often used in the ED for further evaluation of renal pathologies include plain-film abdominal radiography, ultrasound, and CT scan. Plain-film abdominal radiography (KUB, kidneys, ureters, and bladder) is of limited use by itself. It may show the presence of renal calculi or gas; however, the sensitivity is lower than that of CT scan and does not demonstrate complications such as obstruction or hydronephrosis [31]. Plain-film abdominal radiography (KUB film) is useful for the rapid evaluation of urinary stent position.

Emergency physicians are becoming more familiar with the use of renal ultrasound. Emergency medicine residency programs have now included ultrasound training within their curriculum. Renal ultrasound is a valuable diagnostic tool for the evaluation of acute flank pain, especially in unstable patients who cannot tolerate other diagnostic tests such as CT scan [32–34]. It can be performed at the bedside, is non-invasive, does not involve irradiation, and can provide valuable clinical information immediately. Ultrasound can reveal complications such as hydronephrosis, renal or extrarenal abscesses, and distal hydroureter (eg, ureterovesical or uteropelvic junction). In comparison with CT scan, renal ultrasound is not a good test for the detection of urinary stones or the evaluation of upper and midureter dilatations.

Helical CT scan, in contrast to renal ultrasound, provides more detailed information and is considered the imaging modality of choice for most renal pathologies in the evaluation of flank pain [35–39]. Noncontrast CT scan accurately localizes the size of urinary calculi, hydroureter at all levels, hydronephrosis, gas, and abscess. The precise localization of gas has important therapeutic and prognostic implications and is crucial for the differentiation of emphysematous pyelonephritis from other conditions such as emphysematous pyelitis, perinephric emphysema, or abscess [40–42]. The addition of contrast better enables the delineation of abscess from other structures and can provide insight into renal perfusion and reveal renal infarction, renal artery occlusion, or renal vein thrombosis.

In most instances, especially in young women with uncomplicated infections evidenced by history and physical examination, routine radiographic evaluation is not warranted [43]. Underlying structural abnormalities are uncommon, and focal complications rarely occur in this population. However, imaging studies may provide insight as to the cause of the symptoms (eg, kidney stone with or without infection) in situations in which diagnostic uncertainty exists (eg, moderate-to-severe illness with low degree of pyuria), or in patients who have failed therapy or present with recurrent infections [44]. Imaging studies are especially valuable in identifying patients who may have lesions requiring surgical correction (eg, renal or extra renal abscess, emphysematous pyelonephritis, obstruction).

Early and expedited imaging studies are also recommended in patients who present with UTIs associated with severe sepsis/septic shock. Source control is an essential component of therapy in patients with severe sepsis/septic shock [45]. The clinical diagnosis of complications associated with UTI that requires surgical intervention (eg, obstruction, abscess, emphysematous pyelonephritis) can be difficult, and imaging studies can provide substantial clinical utility in revealing these conditions.

There are no specific formal guidelines for the use of imaging modalities when encountering a patient with UTI. Some investigators have recommended routinely imaging all patients with pyelonephritis who require hospital admission [46]. Although this recommendation may be applicable to severely ill patients, the clinical utility and cost effectiveness of performing routine imaging in all patients with pyelonephritis needs further prospective evaluation. In practice, the decision to perform an imaging study in the UTI setting is most often based on the physician's clinical suspicion of the presence of underlying structural abnormality or other complicating factors (eg, renal or extra renal abscess, urolithiasis, emphysematous pyelonephritis, pyonephrosis). However, for patients with severe illness, the clinical diagnosis of such complications is insufficiently accurate and urgent radiographic evaluation is recommended.

Antimicrobial therapy

The choice of initial empiric antimicrobial therapy depends on a combination of several factors such as patient characteristics (eg, age, gender, pregnancy status, prior history of UTI), infection type (ie, complicated versus uncomplicated), knowledge of the most likely microbiologic etiology and local susceptibility patterns, severity of the condition, cost of therapy, and hospital formulary. Tables 1 and 2 depict recommended antimicrobial therapy in patients with uncomplicated and complicated UTIs, respectively [15,47–49].

Because emergency physicians practice in a hospital environment, they are more likely to be influenced by local hospital antibiograms. However, the over reliance on hospital antibiograms may result in an overestimation of the prevalence of resistance in a community, especially in a condition in which cultures are not routinely obtained (ie, uncomplicated cystitis) [47]. Urine cultures are commonly obtained in older patients, in moderate-to-severe infections, complicated UTIs, immunocompromised individuals, recurrent infections, treatment failures, or those who require hospitalization.

Table 1
Recommended antimicrobial therapy of lower urinary tract infection in adults (recommended dosages are for a 70-kg adult with a normal renal and hepatic function)

Acute uncomplicated cystitis
  Local *E coli* resistance to TMP/SMX < 20% or absence of risk factors for TMP/SMX-
    resistant *E coli* such as diabetes, recent hospitalization, current use of antibiotics, and use
    of TMP/SMX in the previous 3 mo
    – TMP/SMX DS (160/800 mg) 1 tablet bid for 3 d
    – Nitrofurantoin (Macrodantin) 50–100 mg qid for 7 d
    – Nitrofurantoin (Macrobid) 100 mg bid for 7 d
  If *E coli* resistance to TMP/SMX ≥ 20% or presence of risk factors for TMP/SMX-resistant
    E coli such as diabetes, recent hospitalization, current use of antibiotics, and use of TMP/
    SMX in the previous 3 mo
    – Ciprofloxacin 250 mg bid for 3 d
    – Ciprofloxacin ER 500 mg qd for 3 d
    – Levofloxacin 250 mg qd for 3 d
    – Nitrofurantoin (Macrodantin) 50–100 mg qid for 7 d
    – Nitrofurantoin (Macrobid) 100 mg bid for 7 d
    – Cephalexin 500 mg qid for 7 d
Lower urinary tract infection in pregnancy
  – Nitrofurantoin (Macrodantin) 50–100 mg qid for 7 d
  – Nitrofurantoin (Macrobid) 100 mg bid for 7 d
  – Cephalexin 500 mg qid for 7 d
  – Amoxicillin/clavulanate 875/125 mg bid for 7 d
Complicated lower urinary tract infection
  – Ciprofloxacin 250 mg bid for 7 d
  – Ciprofloxacin ER 500 mg qd for 7 d
  – Levofloxacin 250 mg qd for 7 d
  – Amoxicillin/clavulanate 875/125 mg bid for 14 d
  – Cephalexin 500 mg qid for 14 d

  Antimicrobial therapy should be adjusted once culture and susceptibility data are known.
  Abbreviations: DS, double strength; ER, extended release; TMP/SMX, trimethoprim-sulfamethoxazole.

Table 2
Recommended antimicrobial therapy for acute pyelonephritis in adults (recommended dosages
are for a 70-kg adult with a normal renal and hepatic function)

Acute uncomplicated pyelonephritis (outpatient therapy)
 – Ciprofloxacin 500 mg bid for 7 d
 – Ciprofloxacin ER 1000 mg qd for 7 d
 – Levofloxacin 250 mg qd for 7 d
 – Ofloxacin 400 mg bid for 7 d
 – Cephalexin 500 mg qid for 14 d
 – Amoxicillin/clavulanate 875/125 mg bid for 14 d
 – Amoxicillin/clavulanate 500/125 mg tid for 14 d
Acute uncomplicated pyelonephritis (inpatient therapy × 14 d)
 – Ciprofloxacin 400 mg IV bid
 – Levofloxacin 500 mg IV qd
 – Ceftriaxone 1–2 g IV qd
 – Piperacillin/tazobactam 3.375 g IV qid
 – Ticarcillin/clavulanate 3.1 g IV qid
 – Ertapenem 1 g IV qd
 – Ampicillin/sulbactam 3 g IV qid
Severely ill patients (eg, severe sepsis/septic shock)
 – Piperacillin/tazobactam 4.5 g IV tid *plus* Gentamicin 5–7 mg/kg IV qd
Complicated pyelonephritis (eg, catheter related, obstruction, renal transplant, etc; total
  duration of therapy, 2–3 wk)
 – Ciprofloxacin 400 mg IV bid
 – Levofloxacin 500 mg IV qd
 – Piperacillin-tazobactam 3.375 g IV qid
 – Ticarcillin-clavulanate 3.1 g IV qid
 – Imipenem 0.5 g IV qid
 – Meropenem 1 g IV tid
Pyelonephritis in pregnancy (× 14 d)
 – Ceftriaxone 1–2 g IV qd
 – Piperacillin/tazobactam 3.375 g IV qid
 – Ticarcillin/clavulanate 3.1 g IV qid
 – Cephalexin 500 mg qid
 – Amoxicillin/clavulanate 875/125 mg bid

Antimicrobial therapy should be adjusted once culture and susceptibility data are known.
Abbreviations: ER, extended release; IV, intravenous.

These patients are more likely to be infected with resistant organisms [2–5].
In addition, hospital antibiograms do not always provide site-specific pathogen resistance information, and the susceptibility data are often generated
from organisms obtained from a variety of sources (eg, respiratory, urinary,
or intraabdominal, wound infections) [47].

Studies evaluating antimicrobial resistance patterns in patients with UTI
treated in outpatient settings have been hindered by a variety of factors
[50–52]. The limitations of such studies include the source of data (eg, labora-
tory-based survey, retrospective chart review for the diagnosis of UTI), cul-
ture-selection bias, and the absence of culture data for a large proportion of
patients [53]. Susceptibility patterns are dynamic, vary by age and geographic

region, and, to be meaningful, need to be monitored continuously in various outpatient settings (eg, primary care clinics, university clinics).

There are few formal studies that have specifically investigated antimicrobial prescription practice patterns for UTI in the ED [54]. However, evidence from other health care settings (eg, private physicians' offices or hospital clinics) with some of these studies, including EDs, has shown variable prescription practice patterns, most of which do not often follow the current Infectious Disease Society of America (IDSA) guidelines for the treatment of UTIs [50,55,56]. The latest IDSA guidelines on UTI advocate the use of TMP/SMX as first-line therapy for uncomplicated cystitis [57]. However, owing to concerns for the presence of resistance and the potential for clinical failure and its adverse side-effect profile, this drug is not commonly prescribed; instead, fluoroquinolones and oral cephalosporins are more often used [50,55,56].

Antimicrobial resistance is an important issue in UTIs. In studies of TMP/SMX-treated patients with uncomplicated cystitis and acute uncomplicated pyelonephritis, TMP/SMX resistance was associated with greater bacteriologic and clinical failure rates [22,58]. In a retrospective case-control study of 448 ED patients with culture-documented UTI, independent predictors of TMP/SMX resistance were diabetes (odds ratio [OR] 3.1; 95% CI, 1.2, 8.4), recent hospitalization (OR 2.5; 95% CI, 1.1, 5.7), current use of antibiotics (OR 4.5; 95% CI, 2.0, 10.2), and recent use of TMP/SMX (OR 5.1; 95% CI, 2.2, 11.5) [59]. Currently, the recommendation is to avoid TMP/SMX in patients with such risk factors and in areas with at or above 20% TMP/SMX-resistance to *E coli* [47,60].

Commonly administered antimicrobial agents for patients requiring intravenous therapy for the treatment of UTI in the ED include a fluoroquinolone (eg, ciprofloxacin, levofloxacin) or a third-generation cephalosporin (eg, ceftriaxone). Less commonly used drugs may include anti-pseudomonal penicillin (eg, piperacillin/tazobactam, ticarcillin/clavulanate), ampicillin/sulbactam, or ertapenem. In severely ill patients such as those presenting in severe sepsis/septic shock, owing to inconsistent in vitro activity of any one class of antimicrobials, a combination of drugs (eg, piperacillin/tazobactam and gentamicin) is often used to ensure adequate coverage for potential resistant pathogens (eg, *Pseudomonas*, enterococci). Monotherapy with fluoroquinolones (eg, levofloxacin) should be avoided in such patients because of inadequate and inconsistent activity of this class against *Pseudomonas* and enterococcal species.

Urinary tract infection in the presence of indwelling catheter

The diagnosis of UTI in the presence of an indwelling catheter is often challenging, especially in the ED. Depending on the duration of catheterization, most catheterized patients presenting to the ED have bacteriuria often accompanied with pyuria. Hence, on the basis of urinalysis, the distinction between those who are merely colonized and those who have a "true" infection is not straightforward. The diagnosis requires culture and growth of an organism in concentrations greater than 10^2 to 10^3 CFU/mL from a urine specimen collected with a needle from the sampling port of the catheter [61].

In clinical practice, as culture results are not readily available on initial evaluation, emergency physicians rely on the presence of clinical signs and symptoms of infection to diagnose catheter-associated UTI. However, this approach has its pitfalls. Most patients with indwelling urinary catheters who present to the ED are elderly and residing in nursing homes. These patients frequently have multiple medical problems, are on numerous medications, and are usually not able to verbalize their symptoms. In addition, they may lack clinical signs of infection and often present with an altered level of consciousness. Another pitfall is readily attributing signs and symptoms of infection to the urinary source and overlooking other causes of infection (eg, pneumonia, meningitis, ischemic bowel). As catheter-associated UTI is a common cause of nosocomial bacteremia with associated increase in morbidity and mortality [62], empiric antimicrobial therapy, in addition to replacement or removal of the catheter, is often initiated in such patients, especially if no other source of infection is found. These patients often undergo numerous diagnostic studies for evaluation of other potential sources of infection.

Urinary tract infection accompanying urolithiasis

Another challenging clinical situation in the ED is the diagnosis of UTI accompanying urolithiasis, especially when the patient does not have overt signs of infection. In clinical practice, a variable degree of pyuria is frequently encountered in acute presentations of urolithiasis. However, whether this finding reflects nonspecific inflammation or true infection is unclear. In a prospective observational study of 238 adult patients presenting with acute urolithiasis, pyuria was not an accurate indicator of UTI. It exhibited poor sensitivity (52% at a leukocyte threshold of 10 cells/high-power field) and moderate specificity. The risk of infection progressively became elevated as the level of pyuria increased (Table 3) [63].

In practice, owing to the potential for complications (eg, abscess formation, pyonephrosis), most physicians initiate antibiotics in patients with urolithiasis who have pyuria regardless of the presence or absence of clinical signs and symptoms of infection. In a study of patients with pyonephrosis associated with nephrolithiasis, St. Lezin and colleagues [64] found a wide spectrum of clinical presentations, varying from asymptomatic bacteriuria to urosepsis, including patients without fever or peripheral leukocytosis.

Disposition

The majority of patients with UTI are treated in an outpatient setting, including patients with acute pyelonephritis [50]. Referral for ID consultation

Table 3
The predictive value of pyuria at various cut-off points for urinary tract infection accompanying acute urolithiasis

Variable	Sensitivity (95% CI)	Specificity (95% CI)	PPV (95% CI)	NPV (95% CI)
Pyuria	52%	76%	20%	93%
(≥5 cells/HPF)	(32%–72%)	(70%–81%)	(10%–30%)	(89%–97%)
Pyuria	48%	88%	32%	94%
(≥10 cells/HPF)	(28%–68%)	(83%–92%)	(17%–46%)	(90%–97%)
Pyuria	44%	92%	38%	93%
(≥15 cells/HPF)	(25%–63%)	(88%–95%)	(20%–56%)	(90%–97%)
Pyuria	40%	93%	40%	93%
(≥20 cells/HPF)	(21%–59%)	(89%–96%)	(21%–59%)	(90%–96%)

Abbreviations: HPF, high-power field; NPV, negative predictive value; PPV, positive predictive value.

Data from Abrahamian FM, Krishnadasan A, Nguyen C, et al. Pyuria is not an accurate predictor of urinary tract infection accompanying acute urolithiasis [abstract 442]. In: Programs and abstracts of the 44th Annual Meeting of Infectious Disease Society of America. Canada, 2006. p. 131.

is most often requested for complicated cases, or for patients with treatment failures. Even in hospitalized patients, ID specialist consultation is not routine and will most likely involve patients who have a severe infection or a complicated, nonresponding course.

Emergency physicians, unlike ID specialists, encounter UTIs in a wide spectrum of disease severity. In addition, emergency physicians have the frequent experience of encountering patients with worrisome clinical findings (eg, high fever, vomiting, tachycardia) whose symptoms improve or resolve after brief interventions with intravenous fluids, antiemetics, antipyretics, and antibiotics. Such patients may initially appear to be candidates for hospitalization; however, after a brief period of observation and simple interventions, they become suitable for outpatient therapy [65,66]. In a select group of immunocompetent patients who respond to initial treatment and have adequate follow-up and return capabilities, the outpatient treatment of pyelonephritis with oral antibiotics is a safe and cost-effective method of therapy [67]. A common practice in the ED is to administer the first dose of antibiotic intravenously before discharge on oral antibiotics [58,68,69]. If deemed appropriate for discharge, to assess the patient's clinical course, and review the culture and susceptibility tests, it should be recommended or arranged for patients to follow up with their primary provider on an outpatient basis.

The main indications for hospitalization are intractable nausea or vomiting (ie, inability to tolerate fluids), hemodynamic instability (including severe sepsis/septic shock), and the presence of complications (eg, obstruction, emphysematous pyelonephritis). Other reasons for hospitalization may include the existence of concomitant immunocompromised states (eg, diabetes mellitus, cancer), patients with indwelling catheters, failure of outpatient therapy, and poor social support (eg, inability to purchase medications or follow-up, homelessness).

Owing to the potential for both maternal and fetal complications, pregnant patients with pyelonephritis are most often admitted to the hospital (at least for a brief period of observation) and treated aggressively with intravenous antibiotics. Oral outpatient therapy has been shown to be safe and effective for the treatment of acute pyelonephritis during the first and second trimester of pregnancy [70–72]. However, studies investigating outpatient therapy of pyelonephritis in pregnant patients included a short hospitalization period with the initiation of an intravenous antibiotic regimen for 48 hours or until afebrile for 48 hours [71,72]. No outpatient trials have been conducted in pregnant patients in whom oral therapy was used alone.

Summary

Emergency physicians encounter UTIs in a wide spectrum of disease severity and patient populations. In the ED, symptomatic UTIs in adults are often categorized as an uncomplicated UTI (cystitis or pyelonephritis) occurring in a woman versus a complicated UTI occurring in a woman or man. Unusual presentations are common, and some patients may lack the classic symptoms of UTI. The diagnosis is especially challenging in the elderly, those with indwelling catheters, and in patients with concomitant acute urolithiasis. The majority of patients do not require an extensive diagnostic evaluation, and most patients can be safely managed as outpatients with oral antibiotics.

References

[1] Arstila T, Huovinen S, Lager K, et al. Positive correlation between the age of patients and the degree of antimicrobial resistance among urinary strains of *Escherichia coli*. J Infect 1994; 29(1):9–16.
[2] Sotto A, De Boever CM, Fabbro-Peray P, et al. Risk factors for antibiotic-resistant *Escherichia coli* isolated from hospitalized patients with urinary tract infections: a prospective study. J Clin Microbiol 2001;39(2):438–44.
[3] Lepelletier D, Caroff N, Reynaud A, et al. *Escherichia coli*: epidemiology and analysis of risk factors for infections caused by resistant strains. Clin Infect Dis 1999;29(3):548–52.
[4] Ena J, Amador C, Martinez C, et al. Risk factors for acquisition of urinary tract infections caused by ciprofloxacin resistant *Escherichia coli*. J Urol 1995;153(1):117–20.
[5] Wright SW, Wrenn KD, Haynes M, et al. Prevalence and risk factors for multidrug resistant uropathogens in ED patients. Am J Emerg Med 2000;18(2):143–6.
[6] Ronald A. The etiology of urinary tract infection: traditional and emerging pathogens. Dis Mon 2003;49(2):71–82.
[7] Bent S, Nallamothu BK, Simel DL, et al. Does this woman have an acute uncomplicated urinary tract infection? JAMA 2002;287(20):2701–10.
[8] Shapiro T, Dalton M, Hammock J, et al. The prevalence of urinary tract infections and sexually transmitted disease in women with symptoms of a simple urinary tract infection stratified by low colony count criteria. Acad Emerg Med 2005;12(1):38–44.

[9] Huppert JS, Biro F, Lan D, et al. Urinary symptoms in adolescent females: STI or UTI? J Adolesc Health 2007;40(5):418–24.

[10] Huppert JS, Biro FM, Mehrabi J, et al. Urinary tract infection and Chlamydia infection in adolescent females. J Pediatr Adolesc Gynecol 2003;16(3):133–7.

[11] Pinson AG, Philbrick JT, Lindbeck GH, et al. Fever in the clinical diagnosis of acute pyelonephritis. Am J Emerg Med 1997;15(2):148–51.

[12] Harding GK, Marrie TJ, Ronald AR, et al. Urinary tract infection localization in women. JAMA 1978;240(11):1147–51.

[13] Busch R, Huland H. Correlation of symptoms and results of direct bacterial localization in patients with urinary tract infections. J Urol 1984;132(2):282–5.

[14] Walter FG, Knopp RK. Urine sampling in ambulatory women: midstream clean-catch versus catheterization. Ann Emerg Med 1989;18(2):166–72.

[15] Fihn SD. Acute uncomplicated urinary tract infection in women. N Engl J Med 2003;349(3): 259–66.

[16] Lammers RL, Gibson S, Kovacs D, et al. Comparison of test characteristics of urine dipstick and urinalysis at various test cutoff points. Ann Emerg Med 2001;38(5):505–12.

[17] Nys S, van Merode T, Bartelds AI, et al. Urinary tract infections in general practice patients: diagnostic tests versus bacteriological culture. J Antimicrob Chemother 2006; 57(5):955–8.

[18] Kunin CM, White LV, Hua TH. A reassessment of the importance of "low-count" bacteriuria in young women with acute urinary symptoms. Ann Intern Med 1993;119(6):454–60.

[19] Richards D, Toop L, Chambers S, et al. Response to antibiotics of women with symptoms of urinary tract infection but negative dipstick urine test results: double blind randomized controlled trial. BMJ 2005;331(7509):143–6.

[20] Carlson KJ, Mulley AG. Management of acute dysuria. A decision-analysis model of alternative strategies. Ann Intern Med 1985;102(2):244–9.

[21] Schultz HJ, McCaffrey LA, Keys TF, et al. Acute cystitis: a prospective study of laboratory tests and duration of therapy. Mayo Clin Proc 1984;59(6):391–7.

[22] Raz R, Chazan B, Kennes Y, et al. Empiric use of trimethoprim-sulfamethoxazole (TMP-SMX) in the treatment of women with uncomplicated urinary tract infections, in a geographical area with a high prevalence of TMP-SMX-resistant uropathogens. Clin Infect Dis 2002; 34(9):1165–9.

[23] Velasco M, Martinez JA, Moreno-Martinez A, et al. Blood cultures for women with uncomplicated acute pyelonephritis: are they necessary? Clin Infect Dis 2003;37(8):1127–30.

[24] MacMillan MC, Grimes DA. The limited usefulness of urine and blood cultures in treating pyelonephritis in pregnancy. Obstet Gynecol 1991;78(5 Pt 1):745–8.

[25] Wing DA, Park AS, DeBuque L, et al. Limited clinical utility of blood and urine cultures in the treatment of acute pyelonephritis during pregnancy. Am J Obstet Gynecol 2000;182(6): 1437–40.

[26] McMurray BR, Wrenn KD, Wright SW. Usefulness of blood cultures in pyelonephritis. Am J Emerg Med 1997;15(2):137–40.

[27] Thanassi M. Utility of urine and blood cultures in pyelonephritis. Acad Emerg Med 1997; 4(8):797–800.

[28] Chen Y, Nitzan O, Saliba W, et al. Are blood cultures necessary in the management of women with complicated pyelonephritis? J Infect 2006;53(4):235–40.

[29] Pasternak EL, Topinka MA. Blood cultures in pyelonephritis: do results change therapy? Acad Emerg Med 2000;7(10):1170.

[30] Hsu CY, Fang HC, Chou KJ, et al. The clinical impact of bacteremia in complicated acute pyelonephritis. Am J Med Sci 2006;332(4):175–80.

[31] Levine JA, Neitlich J, Verga M, et al. Ureteral calculi in patients with flank pain: correlation of plain radiography with unenhanced helical CT. Radiology 1997;204(1):27–31.

[32] Gaspari RJ, Horst K. Emergency ultrasound and urinalysis in the evaluation of flank pain. Acad Emerg Med 2005;12(12):1180–4.

[33] Kartal M, Eray O, Erdogru T, et al. Prospective validation of a current algorithm including bedside US performed by emergency physicians for patients with acute flank pain suspected for renal colic. Emerg Med J 2006;23(5):341–4.

[34] Henderson SO, Hoffner RJ, Aragona JL, et al. Bedside emergency department ultrasonography plus radiography of the kidneys, ureters, and bladder vs intravenous pyelography in the evaluation of suspected ureteral colic. Acad Emerg Med 1998;5:666–71.

[35] Miller OF, Kane CJ. Unenhanced helical computed tomography in the evaluation of acute flank pain. Curr Opin Urol 2000;10(2):123–9.

[36] Dalrymple NC, Verga M, Anderson KR, et al. The value of unenhanced helical computerized tomography in the management of acute flank pain. J Urol 1998;159(3):735–40.

[37] Jindal G, Ramchandani P. Acute flank pain secondary to urolithiasis: radiologic evaluation and alternate diagnoses. Radiol Clin North Am 2007;45(3):395–410.

[38] Vieweg J, Teh C, Freed K, et al. Unenhanced helical computerized tomography for the evaluation of patients with acute flank pain. J Urol 1998;160(3 Pt 1):679–84.

[39] Sheafor DH, Hertzberg BS, Freed KS, et al. Nonenhanced helical CT and US in the emergency evaluation of patients with renal colic: prospective comparison. Radiology 2000; 217(3):792–7.

[40] Bohlman ME, Sweren BS, Khazan R, et al. Emphysematous pyelitis and emphysematous pyelonephritis characterized by computerized tomography. South Med J 1991;84(12):1438–43.

[41] Evanoff GV, Thompson CS, Foley R, et al. Spectrum of gas within the kidney. Emphysematous pyelonephritis and emphysematous pyelitis. Am J Med 1987;83(1):149–54.

[42] Roy C, Pfleger DD, Tuchmann CM, et al. Emphysematous pyelitis: findings in five patients. Radiology 2001;218(3):647–50.

[43] Johnson JR, Vincent LM, Wang K, et al. Renal ultrasonographic correlates of acute pyelonephritis. Clin Infect Dis 1992;14(1):15–22.

[44] Neal DE, Steele R, Sloane B. Ultrasonography in the differentiation of complicated and uncomplicated acute pyelonephritis. Am J Kidney Dis 1990;16(5):478–80.

[45] Nguyen HB, Rivers EP, Abrahamian FM, et al. Severe sepsis and septic shock: review of the literature and emergency department management guidelines. Ann Emerg Med 2006;48(1): 28–54.

[46] Shen Y, Brown MA. Renal imaging in pyelonephritis. Nephrology 2004;9(1):22–5.

[47] Hooton TM, Besser R, Foxman B, et al. Acute uncomplicated cystitis in an era of increasing antibiotic resistance: a proposed approach to empirical therapy. Clin Infect Dis 2004;39(1): 75–80.

[48] Gilbert DN, Moellering RC, Eliopoulos GM, et al. The Sanford Guide to antimicrobial therapy. 37th edition. Sperryville (VA): Antimicrobial Therapy, Inc.; 2007. p. 29–30.

[49] Nicolle LE. Urinary tract infection: traditional pharmacologic therapies. Dis Mon 2003; 49(2):111–28.

[50] Czaja CA, Scholes D, Hooton TM, et al. Population-based epidemiologic analysis of acute pyelonephritis. Clin Infect Dis 2007;45(3):273–80.

[51] Gupta K, Sahm DF, Mayfield D, et al. Antimicrobial resistance among uropathogens that cause community-acquired urinary tract infections in women: a nationwide analysis. Clin Infect Dis 2001;33(1):89–94.

[52] Karlowsky JA, Kelly LJ, Thornsberry C, et al. Trends in antimicrobial resistance among urinary tract infection isolates of Escherichia coli from female outpatients in the United States. Antimicrob Agents Chemother 2002;46(8):2540–5.

[53] Foxman B, Ki M, Brown P. Antibiotic resistance and pyelonephritis. Clin Infect Dis 2007; 45(3):281–3.

[54] Lautenbach E, Larosa LA, Kasbekar N, et al. Fluoroquinolone utilization in the emergency departments of academic medical centers: prevalence of, and risk factors for, inappropriate use. Arch Intern Med 2003;163(5):601–5.

[55] Taur Y, Smith MA. Adherence to the Infectious Diseases Society of America guidelines in the treatment of uncomplicated urinary tract infection. Clin Infect Dis 2007;44(6):769–74.

[56] Huang ES, Stafford RS. National patterns in the treatment of urinary tract infections in women by ambulatory care physicians. Arch Intern Med 2002;162(1):41–7.

[57] Warren JW, Abrutyn E, Hebel JR, et al. Guidelines for antimicrobial treatment of uncomplicated acute bacterial cystitis and acute pyelonephritis in women. Infectious Diseases Society of America (IDSA). Clin Infect Dis 1999;29(4):745–58.

[58] Talan DA, Stamm WE, Hooton TM, et al. Comparison of ciprofloxacin (7 days) and trimethoprim-sulfamethoxazole (14 days) for acute uncomplicated pyelonephritis in women: a randomized trial. JAMA 2000;283(12):1583–90.

[59] Wright SW, Wrenn KD, Haynes ML. Trimethoprim-sulfamethoxazole resistance among urinary coliform isolates. J Gen Intern Med 1999;14(10):606–9.

[60] Le TP, Miller LG. Empirical therapy for uncomplicated urinary tract infections in an era of increasing antimicrobial resistance: a decision and cost analysis. Clin Infect Dis 2001;33(5): 615–21.

[61] Maki DG, Tambyah PA. Engineering out the risk for infection with urinary catheters. Emerg Infect Dis 2001;7(2):342–7.

[62] Kunin CM, Douthitt S, Dancing J, et al. The association between the use of urinary catheters and morbidity and mortality among elderly patients in nursing homes. Am J Epidemiol 1992; 135(3):291–301.

[63] Abrahamian FM, Krishnadasan A, Nguyen C, et al. Pyuria is not an accurate predictor of urinary tract infection accompanying acute urolithiasis [abstract 442]. Programs and abstracts of the 44th Annual Meeting of Infectious Disease Society of America. Canada, October 2006.

[64] St. Lezin M, Hofmann R, Stoller ML. Pyonephrosis: diagnosis and treatment. Br J Urol 1992;70(4):360–3.

[65] Elkharrat D, Chastang C, Boudiaf M, et al. Relevance in the emergency department of a decisional algorithm for outpatient care of women with acute pyelonephritis. Eur J Emerg Med 1999;6(1):15–20.

[66] Israel RS, Lowenstein SR, Marx JA, et al. Management of acute pyelonephritis in an emergency department observation unit. Ann Emerg Med 1991;20(3):253–7.

[67] Safrin S, Siegel D, Black D. Pyelonephritis in adult women: inpatient versus outpatient therapy. Am J Med 1988;85(6):793–8.

[68] Sanchez M, Collvinent B, Miro O, et al. Short-term effectiveness of ceftriaxone single dose in the initial treatment of acute uncomplicated pyelonephritis in women. A randomized controlled trial. Emerg Med J 2002;19(1):19–22.

[69] Pinson AG, Philbrick JT, Lindbeck GH, et al. ED management of acute pyelonephritis in women: a cohort study. Am J Emerg Med 1994;12(3):271–8.

[70] Angel JL, O'Brien WF, Finan MA, et al. Acute pyelonephritis in pregnancy: a prospective study of oral versus intravenous antibiotic therapy. Obstet Gynecol 1990;76(1):28–32.

[71] Millar LK, Wing DA, Paul RH, et al. Outpatient treatment of pyelonephritis in pregnancy: a randomized controlled trial. Obstet Gynecol 1995;86(4 Pt 1):560–4.

[72] Wing DA, Hendershott CM, Debuque L, et al. Outpatient treatment of acute pyelonephritis in pregnancy after 24 weeks. Obstet Gynecol 1999;94(5 Pt 1):683–8.

ELSEVIER
SAUNDERS

Infect Dis Clin N Am 22 (2008) 89–116

INFECTIOUS
DISEASE CLINICS
OF NORTH AMERICA

Management of Skin and Soft-Tissue Infections in the Emergency Department

Fredrick M. Abrahamian, DO, FACEP[a,b,*],
David A. Talan, MD, FACEP, FAAEM, FIDSA[a,b,c],
Gregory J. Moran, MD, FACEP, FAAEM[a,b,c]

[a]David Geffen School of Medicine at the University of California Los Angeles,
Los Angeles, CA, USA
[b]Department of Emergency Medicine, Olive View–University of California Los Angeles
Medical Center, Sylmar, CA, USA
[c]Department of Medicine, Division of Infectious Diseases, Olive View–University of California
Los Angeles Medical Center, Sylmar, CA, USA

Skin and soft-tissue infections (SSTIs) are among the most common infections encountered by emergency physicians. The spectrum of disease severity as seen by emergency physicians is wide, and can range from mild, uncomplicated cellulitis to cutaneous abscesses and necrotizing SSTIs. Infections can include acute, recurrent, and chronic wounds, and community-associated and health care-associated infections in immunocompetent or immunocompromised hosts.

Because of the nature of their practice, emergency physicians encounter patients on a daily basis with a wide variety of mechanisms that lead to SSTIs. These can include animal and human bites, gunshot wounds, illicit drug injection, work-related injuries, pressure sores, and iatrogenic injuries caused by procedures (eg, intravenous lines). Similarly, infectious disease (ID) specialists see a variety of SSTIs in their practice; however, for the ID specialist the spectrum of disease is more skewed toward patients with a complicated course, those who had multiple treatment failures, and recurrent, severe, or rare and unusual infections. Unlike ID specialists, emergency physicians more frequently have to initiate empiric antibiotics because of the absence of culture and susceptibility results, more often have to consider life

* Corresponding author. Department of Emergency Medicine, Olive View–University of California Los Angeles Medical Center, 14445 Olive View Drive, North Annex, Sylmar, CA 91342-1438.
E-mail address: fmasjc@ucla.edu (F.M. Abrahamian).

0891-5520/08/$ - see front matter © 2008 Elsevier Inc. All rights reserved.
doi:10.1016/j.idc.2007.12.001
id.theclinics.com

and limb-threatening SSTIs, and commonly perform minor surgical care of abscesses and infected wounds.

This article is written from the perspective of the evaluation and initial management of SSTIs in the emergency department (ED). It highlights the management pitfalls and clinical dilemmas pertinent to emergency physicians that are not often encountered by ID specialists. Emphasis is placed on the utility of wound and blood cultures, disposition, methicillin-resistant *Staphylococcus aureus* (MRSA) infections, animal and human bites, and necrotizing SSTIs.

Classification

Numerous classification schemes have been proposed for SSTIs. Each classification divides SSTIs based on specific variables, such as infection of normal skin (primary skin infection) versus infection complicating a chronic skin disorder (secondary infection), acute versus chronic, localized versus diffuse, and nonnecrotizing versus necrotizing infections. Another proposed classification system divides SSTIs based on the severity of local and systemic signs, and symptoms of infection and the presence of comorbidities [1].

The most commonly used classification system for SSTIs is based on the presence or absence of complicating factors (ie, uncomplicated versus complicated infections) [2,3]. This classification system is used by the pharmaceutical industry in the design of registration studies for new antimicrobials.

The Center for Drug Evaluation and Research (CDER) at the United States Food and Drug Administration (FDA) has proposed a series of guidance documents for the pharmaceutical industry in development of antimicrobial drugs for the treatment of SSTIs [3]. According to CDER, the uncomplicated category of SSTI includes simple abscesses, impetiginous lesions, furuncles, and cellulitis. The complicated category includes infections involving deeper skin structures, those requiring formal surgical interventions (eg, infected ulcers, burns, major abscesses), and the presence of a significant underlying medical condition that complicates the response to treatment. Infections involving anaerobic or gram-negative organisms (eg, rectal abscesses) are considered complicated [3]. Table 1 depicts examples of skin infections based on the uncomplicated versus complicated classification scheme [2,3].

The most recent practice guidelines developed by the Infectious Disease Society of America (IDSA) for the diagnosis and management of SSTIs do not categorize skin infections based on the uncomplicated versus complicated terminology [4]. The guidelines are written in reference to specific disease entities (eg, cellulitis, abscess, necrotizing infection), mechanism of injury (eg, animal bites, human bites, infection associated with animal contact, surgical site infection), or host factors (eg, infections in the immunocompromised patient) [4]. Unfortunately, these guidelines were written just as community-associated MRSA (CA-MRSA) was emerging as an

Table 1
Examples of skin and soft-tissue infections based on the uncomplicated versus complicated classification scheme

Uncomplicated infections	Complicated infections
Cellulitis	Traumatic wound infection
Erysipelas	Bite-related wound infection
Abscess, folliculitis, furunculosis	Postoperative wound infection
Impetigo, ecthyma	Secondary infection of a diseased skin (eg, eczema)
	Diabetic foot infection
	Venous stasis ulcers, infected pressure sores
	Perianal skin infection
	Necrotizing infection
	Myonecrosis

Data from DiNubile MJ, Lipsky BA. Complicated infections of skin and skin structures: when the infection is more than skin deep. J Antimicrob Chemother 2004;53(Suppl 2):ii37–50.

important cause of SSTI. The management of SSTIs has changed considerably in the last few years and some of these changes are not reflected in the IDSA guidelines.

Microbiology

The microbiology of SSTIs is dependent on numerous factors, such as the host, the environment (eg, community- versus health care-associated), the mechanism of injury, and the duration and severity of illness. Knowledge of these variables is imperative in the selection of an initial empiric antimicrobial regimen.

In general, *S. aureus,* and to a lesser extent streptococci, are by far the most common causes of both uncomplicated and complicated SSTIs, with a few notable exceptions, such as animal and human bite-wound infections [5,6]. Polymicrobial infections with gram-negative and anaerobic organisms are typically seen in complicated infections [2,5–8].

The most important new development in the era of SSTI is the emergence of CA-MRSA, a phenomenon largely recognized and studied in ED populations. CA-MRSA infections have become a global emerging health problem. Most infections are noninvasive [9], involve skin and soft-tissue structures, and present as purulent skin infections [10–12]. The spectrum of skin infections caused by CA-MRSA is wide and can range from simple cutaneous abscesses to fulminant necrotizing fasciitis [12,13].

In the United States, the most common strain of MRSA associated with community infections is USA300, and less commonly USA400 and USA1000 [12,14]. Compared with health care-associated strains, CA-MRSA strains more frequently produce toxins and appear to be more virulent. The Panton-Valentine leukocidin genes, which produce cytotoxins that cause tissue necrosis, damage host cell membranes, and leukocyte destruction, are commonly seen with CA-MRSA and rarely with health care-associated MRSA (HA-MRSA) strains [15–19]. Novel peptides have been recently identified that are cytotoxic to leukocytes and may be important virulence factors of CA-MRSA [20].

In a recent multicenter, prospective, prevalence study involving adult subjects with purulent SSTIs, MRSA was isolated from 59% of subjects (n = 422; range: 15% to 74%). In this study, MRSA was isolated from 61% of abscesses, 53% of infected wounds, and 47% of cellulitis associated with purulent exudate. Methicillin-susceptible *S. aureus* (MSSA) was isolated from 14% of abscesses, 21% of infected wounds, and 34% of cellulitis associated with purulent exudate. Streptococcal species was isolated from 7% of abscesses, 9% of infected wounds, and 13% of cellulitis associated with purulent exudate [12]. Although it is clear that MRSA is now a common cause of SSTI overall, it is not clear to what extent it is now responsible for all possible subtypes of SSTI, such as diabetic foot infections or bite-wound infections.

In one investigation of ED patients with SSTI, historical and clinical features associated with MRSA compared with other bacteria include a history of close contact with similar infection (odds ratio [OR], 3.4; 95% confidence index or CI, 1.5–8.1; $P < .05$), prior history of MRSA infection (OR, 3.3; 95% CI, 1.2–10.1; $P < .05$), reported "spider bite" (OR, 2.8; 95% CI, 1.5–5.3; $P < .05$), received antibiotics in the past 1 month (OR, 2.4; 95% CI, 1.4–4.1; $P < .05$), and abscess (OR, 1.8; 95% CI, 1.0–3.1; $P < .05$) [12]. A common pitfall is to assume one can reliably exclude MRSA based on the absence of risk factors. However, even in the absence of risk factors, CA-MRSA is still prevalent, and was present in 48% of ED SSTI patients in one investigation [12]. There are no clinical or epidemiologic risk factors that can exclude MRSA etiology and reliably distinguish between patients infected with CA-MRSA and other organisms [11,12,21,22].

Another common mistake is to assume one can also reliably differentiate CA-MRSA and HA-MRSA based on epidemiologic factors. The epidemiologic definition of HA-MRSA infection includes MRSA identified after 48 hours of hospital admission, or identified in patients with a history of surgery, hospitalization, dialysis, or residence in a long-term care facility within the last year, an indwelling catheter or other invasive medical devices, and previous history of MRSA infection or colonization [9,23,24]. The exclusive use of this definition can underestimate the true prevalence of CA-MRSA infection. In the ED-based study by Moran and colleagues [12], almost all MRSA isolated from SSTIs had molecular characteristics of CA-MRSA, even though more than 25% of subjects met the epidemiologic definition of HA-MRSA.

Another pitfall is to assume that pure cellulitis is exclusively caused by streptococci, as suggested by the recent IDSA guidelines [4]. Investigations into the etiology of cellulitis without drainage are limited by the lack of specimen availability. Studies using tissue biopsies and aspirate specimens, and relying on conventional and nonconventional identification methods, such as immunofluorescence and serologic testing, suggest that *S. aureus*—and to much lesser extent streptococci—are the most common pathogens implicated in the pathogenesis of cellulitis [25–32]. With the emergence of CA-MRSA, the role of this pathogen in these difficult-to-study infections is uncertain. In the ED-based study by Moran and colleagues, among cellulitis cases accompanied by purulent drainage, MRSA was found in 47% [12]. Thus, it is reasonable to assume CA-MRSA has a role in these infections. Also, it has become evident that many occult cutaneous abscesses, which are now predominantly caused by CA-MRSA, are misdiagnosed as cellulitis on clinical evaluation, potentially leading to treatment failure, and their detection is greatly enhanced with the use of bedside soft-tissue ultrasonography [33,34].

Necrotizing fasciitis and myonecrosis are typically caused by infection with Group A streptococcus, *Clostridium perfringens*, or, most commonly, aerobic and anaerobic organisms as part of a polymicrobial infection that may include *S. aureus*. In case series, CA-MRSA has recently been described as a predominantly monomicrobial cause of necrotizing fasciitis [35,36]. A retrospective review of patients presenting with necrotizing fasciitis between 2000 and 2006 indicated that MRSA was the most common pathogen, accounting for one-third of the organisms isolated [37].

Other important causes of SSTI, including dog, cat, and human bite infections have been investigated among ED patients. Bite-wound infections are often mixed aerobic and anaerobic infections, with some unique pathogens transmitted by the biter's oral flora. In a study of 107 subjects with dog and cat bite infections, mixed aerobic and anaerobic infections were present in 56% of all wounds (dogs: 48%; cats: 63%) [5]. *Pasteurella* species was the most common pathogen isolated from both dog (50%) and cat (75%) bites and was commonly isolated from abscesses and puncture wounds. The most common pasteurella strain isolated from infected dog bites was *P. canis* (26%), while in infected cat bites it was *P. multocida* subspecies *multocida* (54%). Streptococci were seen in 46% of both types of bite infections. *S. aureus* (all MSSA) was only isolated in 20% of dog bite infections and 4% of cat bite infections, suggesting animal oral flora dominates human skin flora, especially for deep puncture wounds. Anaerobes (eg, *Fusobacterium nucleatum, Bacteroides tectum, Porphyromonas* species, *Prevotella heparinolytica*) were usually present as mixed infections with aerobic organisms.

Similar to animal bites, human bites are also frequently mixed aerobic and anaerobic infections. In a study of 50 subjects with infected human bites, 54% of wounds were mixed aerobic and anaerobic infection with organisms [6]. The most common organisms recovered from human bite wounds included *Streptococcus* species (84%; *S. anginosus* was the most common pathogen, isolated in 52% of cases), *S. aureus* (30%), *Eikenella corrodens* (30%), *Prevotella* species (36%), *Fusobacterium* species (34%), and *Veillonella* species (24%) [6].

Mixed aerobic and anaerobic bacteria are also commonly observed in SSTIs among injecting-drug users (IDUs). A comparative microbiologic study of cutaneous abscesses among IDUs and non-IDUs found a greater frequency of mixed aerobic and anaerobic infections in IDUs. The prevalence of oral anaerobic organisms was higher among IDUs. In addition to *S. aureus*, which was found in 50% of IDU abscess cases, *Streptococcus milleri*, *F. nucleatum*, *Prevotella* species, *Peptostreptococcus micros*, *Actinomyces odontolyticus*, and *Veillonella* species were found [38].

Clinical presentation

The clinical manifestations of SSTIs are variable and depends on factors such as the host, the infecting organism, and the inciting event. CA-MRSA SSTIs commonly present as a spontaneous abscess [10–12]. The patient often attributes the infection to a "spider bite." Misclassification of a deep abscess as cellulitis is a common pitfall. Physicians often attribute treatment failure of "cellulitis" to antimicrobial resistance and change to a different, or often multiple, antibiotic regimen. The presence of an underlying deep abscess should be considered in patients with cellulitis who "fail" initial antimicrobial therapy. Treatment failure may be caused by an undrained abscess that was missed on the initial presentation, rather than inadequate antimicrobial therapy. Bedside ultrasound is more frequently available in the ED and is recommended for evaluation of all suspicious SSTIs.

Some wounds may be associated with injuries to deeper structures, such as bones, joints, tendons, and neurovascular structures. Animal and human bite injuries that appear to be minor may have underlying joint and other structural injuries. Clenched fist injuries ("fight bites") are particularly prone to underlying bone or metacarpal joint involvement that can be missed on initial presentation. Cats, with their sharp thin teeth, often produce small deep puncture wounds that seem to be trivial, but further evaluation may reveal joint or cortical injuries. Pain out of proportion to the wound and physical findings should raise suspicion for joint or bony injuries.

Different terms and classifications have been used to describe various types of necrotizing SSTIs (eg, synergistic necrotizing cellulitis, necrotizing fasciitis, streptococcal myonecrosis, gas gangrene). Although various factors may distinguish each type of infection, it is currently recommended to describe these generally as "necrotizing soft-tissue infections" or necrotizing SSTI, because their initial treatment, which emphasizes early surgical intervention and broad-spectrum antimicrobials, is the same [39].

Patients with necrotizing SSTI most often present with severe pain (often out of proportion to physical findings) and rapidly advancing induration and tenderness that extends beyond the area of erythema. These patients appear ill and most often have abnormal vital signs on presentation. However, the recognition of a necrotizing SSTI, especially in the early stages, is extremely difficult. Patients present in variable stages in the spectrum of the illness. In a retrospective review of 89 patients with necrotizing fasciitis, only 13 (15%) patients had the diagnosis of necrotizing fasciitis at the time of admission [35]. At the time of the presentation, patients can be afebrile [36,40] and have minimal pain at the site of infection [36]. The cutaneous findings early in the course of disease may be lacking or are nonspecific. In a retrospective review of patients with necrotizing SSTIs, the most specific signs, crepitus and blistering, were absent in 63% (n = 189) and 76% (n = 190) of patients, respectively [40]. In 15% of patients (n = 170), none of the specific findings, (ie, crepitus, blistering, or radiographic evidence of soft-tissue gas) were present [40]. Lymphangitis and lymphadenopathy are typically absent [41].

Recent reports (mostly case reports and case series) of necrotizing SSTIs caused by CA-MRSA have revealed that this type of necrotizing SSTI presents more subacutely and is a more benign syndrome than necrotizing infections caused by other etiologies [13,42–44]. In a retrospective study of 14 patients with necrotizing SSTIs, 57% of patients had a preoperative diagnosis of abscess, and necrotizing infection was not suspected [13]. In this series, the onset of disease was often subacute (average 6 days; range, 3–21), and even in the presence of serious complications (eg, need for reconstructive surgery and prolonged stay in the intensive care unit), none of the patients died [13]. The 100% survival rate in this series, compared with the approximately 70% survival in most necrotizing SSTI series [36,40], suggests that perhaps some of these may be a different type of necrotizing infection. Large abscesses that can be caused by CA-MRSA are sometimes found to have necrotic tissue, even though they are not associated with the high mortality of what has been traditionally considered to be a necrotizing infection.

Laboratory evaluation and imaging

Microbiologic studies, such as wound cultures and blood cultures, can be of value in selected patients with SSTIs; however, their routine use in all SSTI is debated [45]. Historically, routine wound cultures were rarely performed because of the predictable infection etiology and the associated antimicrobial susceptibility patterns. In the current era of increased prevalence of SSTIs caused by CA-MRSA, and varying antimicrobial susceptibility patterns—even among CA-MRSA strains—more physicians are performing wound cultures to assess the etiology of the infection and guide further antimicrobial therapy.

The decision to do any diagnostic test, including wound or blood cultures, depends on its clinical utility and the likelihood that the result will change management. The majority of patients with CA-MRSA infection will present with simple, uncomplicated abscess [12]. Although the additional benefit of CA-MRSA active antibiotics requires further study, based on the current available evidence, the management of uncomplicated abscesses, even those caused by CA-MRSA, is solely incision and drainage, which is associated with a cure rate of 85% to 90% [12,46–48]. Therefore, it is unlikely that culture and susceptibility testing would be helpful in the patient's care.

Wound cultures should be reserved for patients that have a greater chance of treatment failure, such as patients with complicated infections, immunocompromising conditions, moderate-to-severe illness, refractory or recurrent infections, and those that have failed prior surgical therapy. Wound cultures are also appropriate for patients who will be treated with an antibiotic with variable activity against the presumed pathogen (eg, CA-MRSA and clindamycin). Cultures should be obtained for all patients admitted to the hospital, both to ensure that the empiric regimen has activity against the pathogen, and to allow appropriate narrowing of the antimicrobial spectrum (eg, switch vancomycin to oxacillin if MSSA is identified).

Although pathogen prevalence rates and susceptibility patterns can be surmised from the selected group of patients who require cultures, broader local surveillance can help to determine optimal empiric therapy for future patients. However, patients should be spared the expense of tests for which they receive no direct benefit, and costs of surveillance testing should be borne by public health departments or health care systems. At this point in time, CA-MRSA appears to be a frequent and endemic cause of SSTI; however, its antimicrobial susceptibility pattern appears to be changing.

As with wound cultures, the utility of blood cultures in all types of SSTIs is also debated. A typical case of a cellulitis deemed appropriate for outpatient antimicrobial therapy is unlikely to be associated with bacteremia. Even for hospitalized patients with community-acquired cellulitis, bacteremia is an uncommon finding [49], and discordant antibiotic therapy is rare. In a study of 757 hospitalized subjects with community-acquired cellulitis [49], blood cultures were performed on 553 subjects. A "true" pathogen (ie, not a contaminant) was isolated from the blood cultures in only 11 cases (2%) [49]. In order of decreasing frequency, isolated organisms included: Group G streptococcus (5), Group A streptococcus (3), S. aureus (1), Vibrio vulnificus (1), and Morganella morganii (1). Univariate regression analysis revealed that an age greater than 45 years, short duration of symptoms before presentation, temperature higher or equal to 38.5°C, and white blood cell (WBC) count greater than 13,300/mm^3 at admission were predictive of bacteremia. Initial empiric antimicrobial therapy was concordant in all patients with bacteremia. For the two patients with gram-negative bacteremia, there was sufficient historical information to suspect an infection with an unusual organism. One patient with V. vulnificus bacteremia was a 69-year-old male, with a history of fish bone injury to his right hand second digit, who developed cellulitis and chills 6 hours after the injury. Another patient with M. morganii bacteremia was a 50-year-old female with past medical history of noninsulin-dependent diabetes mellitus and end-stage renal disease, receiving hemodialysis that was temporality administered through an indwelling central catheter. Contaminated samples were almost twice as common as true-positive blood cultures. False-positive blood culture results have the potential for introducing inappropriate treatment and can increase length of hospital stay, resource use, and costs [50].

The latest IDSA SSTI guidelines [4] mention the low yield of blood cultures; however, they fail to clearly recommend which patients would benefit from them. Other sources recommend reserving blood cultures for patients with signs and symptoms of systemic toxicity, severe infections, those with chills and high-grade fever, elderly patients with acute onset of illness, significant leukocytosis, and immunocompromised patients [1,4,49,51]. However, most patients that are considered for hospitalization have some to all of these loosely defined criteria.

Blood cultures are only helpful if the results would identify the need for a change in a patient's therapy such that it would improve clinical outcomes. ID specialists should reconsider the need for routine blood cultures in ED patients who are to be admitted to the hospital with SSTI, especially if the pathogen can be isolated from the infected wound or abscess. Instances in which blood cultures could be of clinical utility can include patients with SSTI who present with severe sepsis or septic shock [52], are at risk for an unusual infection requiring unusual therapy, have immunocompromising conditions, and for whom the finding of bacteremia would have important implications, such as patients at risk for endovascular infection (eg, those with prosthetic heart valves).

Other diagnostic tests to investigate the microbiologic etiology of SSTIs have included cultures from needle aspirations of inflamed skin (either at the point of maximal inflammation or the leading edge) and tissue punch biopsies. The positive yields of these techniques are variable and, overall, low [25–28,53], and as a result are not recommended.

Tissue biopsy and frozen section examination has been advocated for patients with suspected necrotizing SSTI [54,55]. However, correct interpretation of this test requires an experienced pathologist (not often available at all times), and the process can result in a delay in surgical intervention. Most surgeons prefer to explore the site of infection directly in the operating room. Rapid streptococcal antigen testing of the wound (which is only approved for pharyngeal infections) in the ED has been reported to provide early identification of streptococcal toxic shock syndrome [56]. Serologic tests for streptococcal infection are not helpful in the ED because meaningful interpretation of these tests requires paired acute and convalescent titers.

Basic hematologic studies and serum chemistries are commonly performed on patients requiring hospital admission. These tests can aid in assessing the severity of disease, reveal organ dysfunction, and may expose underlying medical conditions (eg, anemia, renal disease). The most recent IDSA SSTI guidelines recommend obtaining these tests in patients with signs and symptoms of systemic toxicity (eg, fever, hypothermia, tachycardia, and hypotension) [4].

A diagnostic scoring system based on laboratory tests has been proposed as a tool for distinguishing necrotizing SSTI from other SSTIs [57]. The Laboratory Risk Indicator for Necrotizing Fasciitis (LRINEC) score is depicted in Table 2. The score assigns points based on the level of various laboratory variables that include C-reactive protein, total WBC count, serum sodium, creatinine, glucose, and hemoglobin. The maximum cumulative score is 13. A score greater than or equal to 6 had a positive predictive value of 92% (95% CI, 84.3–96.0) and negative predictive value of 96% (95% CI, 92.6–97.9) for necrotizing SSTI. The probability of necrotizing SSTI increased to more than 75% when the LRINEC score was greater than or equal to 8 (Table 3). The authors advocate using this tool as an adjunct in the management of SSTI. However, the ability of the LRINEC score to detect early cases of necrotizing SSTI is unproven.

The derivation of the LRINEC score was based on a retrospective observational study of subjects divided into developmental or derivation (n = 314) and validation (n = 140) cohorts [57]. Because of the retrospective nature of the study, for both groups (developmental and validation cohorts) the diagnosis of necrotizing SSTI and nonnecrotizing SSTI was already made. Unfortunately, the utility of the LRINEC score is potentially limited

Table 2
Laboratory Risk Indicator for Necrotizing Fasciitis score

Laboratory parameter (units)	LRINEC points
C-reactive protein (mg/L)	
<150	0
≥150	4
Total white blood cell count (mm^3)	
<15	0
15–25	1
>25	2
Hemoglobin (g/dL)	
>13.5	0
11–13.5	1
<11	2
Sodium (mmol/L)	
≥135	0
<135	2
Creatinine (mg/dL)	
≤1.6	0
>1.6	2
Glucose (mg/dL)	
≤180	0
>180	1

Modified from Wong CH, Khin LW, Heng KS, et al. The LRINEC (Laboratory Risk Indicator for Necrotizing Fasciitis) score: a tool for distinguishing necrotizing fasciitis from other soft- tissue infections. Crit Care Med 2004;32(7):1535–41; with permission.

Table 3
Laboratory Risk Indicator for Necrotizing Fasciitis score and the corresponding risk category and probability of necrotizing skin and soft-tissue infection

LRINEC score	Risk category	Probability of necrotizing skin and soft-tissue infection
≤ 5	Low	< 50%
6–7	Intermediate	50%–75%
≥ 8	High	> 75%

Modified from Anaya DA, Dellinger EP. Necrotizing soft-tissue infection: diagnosis and management. Clin Infect Dis 2007;44(5):705–10; with permission.

in that it needs to be prospectively validated in patients for whom the diagnosis of necrotizing SSTI is not apparent on initial history and physical examination, thus testing the ability of the score to detect early and atypical presentations that would benefit from earlier surgical intervention.

It is also unclear if the LRINEC score can be applied to all age groups. The youngest subjects enrolled in the developmental and validation cohorts were 27 and 13 years of age, respectively [57]. C-reactive protein, a test component of LRINEC score, is also not a universally available test and has a variable turn-around time; hence, its utility is somewhat limited. However, finding abnormalities that make up the LRINEC score in patients with SSTI should increase suspicion of a necrotizing infection such that further observation and evaluation should be considered. Although not part of the LRINEC score, an elevated creatine kinase should also increase suspicion of a necrotizing infection. Urinalysis can provide a clue to the presence of rhabdomyolysis by demonstrating blood in urine in the absence of red blood cells.

Other diagnostic tests used in the evaluation of SSTIs include soft-tissue radiographs, CT scans, ultrasonography, and magnetic resonance imaging. Utilization of these adjunctive diagnostic tests is based upon the physician's index of suspicion for osteomyelitis, subcutaneous emphysema, or deep abscess. However, it is also important to understand the limitations of these tests. In a study of 148 subjects with necrotizing SSTI, 27% of subjects did not have evidence of soft-tissue gas in plain radiographs or CT scans [40]. In another study, only 29% (n = 65) of subjects had evidence of soft-tissue gas in plain radiographs or CT scans [36].

Ultrasonography can be useful in the identification of deep abscesses, especially in cases in which the physical examination is equivocal or there is a broad area of what appears to be cellulitis. In this situation, ultrasound has been shown to have greater sensitivity and specificity in detecting deep abscesses than clinical examination alone (sensitivity: 98% versus 86%; specificity: 88% versus 70%) [33,34].

Drainage and debridement

Incision and drainage is a commonly performed procedure to treat cutaneous abscesses and emergency physicians are very familiar with performing this procedure. A step-by-step, descriptive video clip of how to perform incision and drainage can be viewed at http://content.nejm.org/cgi/content/short/357/19/e20 [58].

The initial step in performing an incision and drainage is to prepare the site for incision and remove any dirt or debris. The infected area is further cleaned with a skin-cleansing agent (eg, chlorhexidine, povidone iodine, or isopropyl alcohol). Although this procedure is not considered sterile, the physician should attempt to keep the area as clean as possible and devoid of unnecessary contamination.

The area is anesthetized with preservative-free 1% to 2% lidocaine. Injection of lidocaine within the abscess cavity has not been shown to alter microbiologic data [59]. After 2 to 5 minutes, when the onset of anesthesia has occurred, using a number 11 scalpel, a straight incision is made over the area of maximal fluctuance. The length of the incision will depend on the size of the abscess; however, in general, the incision ought to be made large enough to promote adequate drainage. After obtaining culture material (if indicated) and the initial decompression of purulent material, the abscess cavity is probed thoroughly using a curved or straight hemostat. This action will further release any pockets of purulent material and break any remaining loculations and adhesions. All necrotic and devitalized tissue is also debrided.

To remove all loosened purulent and necrotic material, the abscess cavity is irrigated with sterile saline, using an 18-gauge angiocatheter attached to a 10-mL syringe. Although it is recommended [58], the additional clinical utility of irrigating the abscess cavity is unknown.

After thorough drainage and removal of purulent material and any devitalized tissue, the abscess cavity is loosely packed using $\frac{1}{4}$ - or $\frac{1}{2}$ -inch plain packing strips. In order to ensure that the incision site will remain open and allow for continued drainage, 1 cm to 2 cm of the packing material is left extending outside of the wound. The last step involves covering the wound with absorbent 4 × 4 gauze dressing. Patients are instructed to return within a few days for removal of the packing material, or can be instructed to change the packing themselves at home. Some patients will need a prescription of narcotic analgesic for dressing changes.

Antimicrobial therapy

The choice of initial empiric antimicrobial therapy is dependent upon prediction of the most likely microbiologic etiology and local antimicrobial susceptibility patterns. Table 4 depicts recommended initial empiric antimicrobial therapy options for commonly encountered SSTIs in the ED.

The mechanism of injury is crucial to predicting the bacterial etiology, which is especially important if organisms are involved that require specific treatment. Examples of acute infections in which mechanism of injury is key include dog and cat bite infections (*Pasteurella* species), human bite infections (*Eikenella* species), salt-water (*Vibrio* species) and fresh-water (*Aeromonas* species) exposure.

CA-MRSA is the most common cause of purulent SSTIs in most areas of the United States [12]. It demonstrates variable susceptibility patterns to commonly used agents, such as clindamycin and tetracyclines. In vitro susceptibility patterns of CA-MRSA to a variety of antimicrobial agents are depicted in Table 5 [12,21,23,60]. Antibiotics that have adequate activity against CA-MRSA include trimethoprim/sulfamethoxazole (TMP/SMX), rifampin, vancomycin, linezolid (Zyvox), daptomycin (Cubicin), tigecycline (Tygacil), and quinupristin-dalfopristin (Synercid) [12,21,23,60–68].

Currently, the clinical trials for off-patent antibiotics for uncomplicated SSTIs are being planned with support of the National Institutes of Health. Other potential future MRSA antimicrobials that are currently in various phases of clinical trials for SSTI include novel glycopeptides, such as dalbavancin (administered once weekly), telavancin, oritavancin (LY333328), ceftobiprole (a cephalosporin with anti-MRSA activity), and Iclaprim (formerly AR-100, Ro 48-2622; a specific and selective microbial dihydrofolate reductase inhibitor) [69–73].

The most common type of SSTI associated with CA-MRSA is an abscess [10–12,47,60]. Although further study is needed to determine if antibiotics lead to additional benefit for CA-MRSA abscesses, it appears that 85% to 90% of patients do well with a treatment of incision and drainage alone [12,46–48]. In a recent observational study of 492 adult patients with CA-MRSA SSTIs, the use of an inactive antimicrobial agent was found to be an independent predictor of treatment failure (adjusted OR, 2.80; 95% CI, 1.26–6.22; $P = .01$) [60]. However, of the 45 patients who experienced treatment failure, 38 (84%) were attributed to the need for additional incision and drainage.

In an observational study of 69 children with culture-proven CA-MRSA abscesses, a patient with an abscess greater than or equal to 5 cm in diameter was more likely to require subsequent hospitalization with incision and drainage alone [46]. Based on this study, The Sanford Guide recommends instituting antibiotics for patients with abscesses greater than or equal to 5 cm in diameter [74]. Unfortunately, these findings derive from observational data in which the incision and drainage procedure was not standardized. In the authors' experience, the most common reason abscesses fail initial management is inadequate incision and drainage, irrespective of the activity of the antibiotic against CA-MRSA, and inadequate drainage is more likely with larger abscesses if there is not careful attention to proper technique.

In the absence of large randomized trials conducted in the area of CA-MRSA, current recommendations on antimicrobial therapy of CA-MRSA SSTIs are based on expert opinion [24]. In conjunction with surgical drainage, the IDSA SSTI guidelines recommend the addition of systemic antimicrobial agents in patients with cutaneous abscesses in the following

Table 4
Recommended initial empiric antimicrobial therapy options for commonly encountered skin
and soft-tissue infections in the emergency department

Infection	Therapeutic setting	Initial empiric antimicrobial therapy
Mild cellulitis	Outpatient therapy	• TMP/SMX DS (160/800 mg) 1–2 tablets bid plus Cephalexin 500 mg qid • Clindamycin 300 mg qid • Minocycline 100 mg bid (first dose, 200 mg) • Doxycycline 100 mg bid
Abscess with mild cellulitis	Outpatient therapy	• Incision and drainage (no need for antimicrobial therapy). • Use of outpatient antimicrobial therapy is recommended in patients with multiple lesions, immunocompromised state, those with evidence of mild systemic toxicity (eg, fever), recurrent infections, those who have failed initial surgical therapy (after exclusion of inadequate drainage or deeper abscess), and abscesses that cannot be completely drained. TMP/SMX DS (160/800 mg) 1–2 tablets bid Clindamycin 300 mg qid Minocycline 100 mg bid (first dose, 200 mg) Doxycycline 100 mg bid
Moderate-to-severe cellulitis or abscess	Inpatient parenteral therapy	• Clindamycin 600 mg–900 mg IV q 8 h Monotherapy with clindamycin is preferred only for moderate infections. • Vancomycin 1 g IV q 12 h ± cefazolin 1 g IV q 6 h May replace cefazolin with nafcillin or oxacillin 1 g–2 g every 4 hours. Addition of β-lactam agent may provide enhanced activity against MSSA or streptococci (preferred for patients suspected to be bacteremic with *S. aureus*).
Diabetic foot infection	Outpatient therapy	• Clindamycin 300 mg qid plus Ciprofloxacin 500 mg bid • Amoxicillin/clavulanate 875/125 mg bid ± TMP/SMX DS (160/800 mg) 1–2 tablets bid

(*continued on next page*)

Table 4 (*continued*)

Infection	Therapeutic setting	Initial empiric antimicrobial therapy
Diabetic foot infection	Inpatient parenteral therapy	• Ceftriaxone 1 g IV q 24 h plus metronidazole 500 mg IV q 6–8 h ± Vancomycin 1 g IV q 12 h • Ertapenem 1 g IV q 24 h ± vancomycin 1 g IV q 12 h • Tigecycline 50 mg IV q 12 h (first dose, 100 mg IV)
Dog, cat, and human bites	Outpatient therapy	• Amoxicillin/clavulanate 875/125 mg bid • Moxifloxacin 400 mg daily • Clindamycin 300 mg qid plus Ciprofloxacin 500 mg bid
Dog, cat, and human bites	Inpatient parenteral therapy	• Ampicillin/sulbactam 1.5 g–3 g IV q 6 h • Moxifloxacin 400 mg IV qd
Necrotizing soft-tissue infections		• Vancomycin 1 g IV q 12 h plus Clindamycin 900 mg IV q 8 h plus Piperacillin/ tazobactam 3.375 g IV q 6 h May replace vancomycin with daptomycin 4 mg/kg–6 mg/kg IV qd. Clindamycin (or alternatively linezolid, see below) is recommended because of its ability to inhibit toxin production. May substitute piperacillin/tazobactam with imipenem or meropenem. • Linezolid 600 mg IV q 12 h plus Piperacillin/tazobactam 3.375 g IV q 6 h

Recommended dosages are for a non-pregnant 70-kg adult with a normal renal and hepatic function. Antimicrobial therapy should be initiated based on knowledge of local susceptibility patterns and adjusted once culture and susceptibility data are known.

Abbreviations: DS, double-strength; IV, intravenous; TMP/SMX, trimethoprim-sulfamethoxazole.

situations: multiple lesions, cutaneous gangrene, immunocompromised state, extensive surrounding cellulitis, and those with evidence of systemic toxicity (eg, high fever) [4]. The initiation of antibiotics is also reasonable in patients requiring hospitalization (a reflection of the severity of the disease), recurrent infections, those who have failed initial surgical therapy (after exclusion of inadequate drainage or deeper abscess), and in abscesses associated with unusual pathogens (eg, human bite).

TMP/SMX is a commonly used drug in the United States for outpatient management of CA-MRSA SSTIs. The Sanford Guide recommends two double-strength TMP/SMX tablets twice a day, with the goal of ensuring

Table 5
In vitro susceptibility patterns of community-associated methicillin-resistant *Staphylococcus aureus* to a variety of antimicrobial agents

Antibiotic	Moran et al [12]	Miller et al [21]	Naimi et al [23]	Ruhe et al [60]
TMP/SMX	100% (n = 217)	100% (n = 120)	95% (n = 106)	99% (n = 322)
Rifampin	100% (n = 186)	100% (n = 120)	96% (n = 106)	99% (n = 318)
Clindamycin	95% (n = 226)[a]	95% (n = 102)	83% (n = 106)	98% (n = 482)[b]
Tetracycline	92% (n = 226)	81% (n = 120)	92% (n = 106)	93% (n = 455)
Gentamicin	NT	100% (n = 120)	94% (n = 106)	100% (n = 320)
Ciprofloxacin	60% (n = 176)	15% (n = 101)	79% (n = 106)	73% (n = 354)
Erythromycin	6% (n = 226)	7% (n = 120)	44% (n = 106)	5% (n = 23)
Vancomycin	NT	100% (n = 120)	100% (n = 106)	100% (n = 492)
Linezolid	NT	100% (n = 19)	NT	NT

Susceptibility patterns are dynamic and may vary markedly by geographic regions. Physicians' familiarity with the prevalence and susceptibility patterns of CA-MRSA in their community is a crucial element in the management of CA-MRSA infections.

Abbreviations: NT, Not tested; TMP/SMX, Trimethoprim/sulfamethoxazole.

[a] Four (approximately 2%; n = 226) MRSA isolates had inducible clindamycin resistance detected by an antimicrobial susceptibility D-zone disk diffusion test.

[b] Two (3%; n = 59) MRSA isolates had inducible clindamycin resistance detected by an antimicrobial susceptibility D-zone disk diffusion test.

Modified from Abrahamian FM, Snyder EW. Community-associated methicillin-resistant *Staphylococcus aureus*: incidence, clinical presentation, and treatment decisions. Curr Infect Dis Rep 2007;9(5):391–7; with permission.

adequate serum levels with respect to the minimum inhibitory concentration (MIC) and maximizing concentration-dependent killing [74]. Although this recommendation seems logical and is made to prevent under-dosing, it should be noted that there are no prospective human trials demonstrating the superiority of a two double-strength, compared with a one double-strength, regimen. TMP/SMX has been shown to have adequate penetration into experimentally made human skin blisters [75,76]; however, the same may not apply to abscesses even with an increased dosage regimen. Most importantly, the issue of penetration into the abscess cavity may be a moot point if they are treated with adequate incision and drainage. Dosage increases may also lead to increased side-effects and potentially lower patient compliance with the advocated regimen.

Rifampin, a highly active agent against CA-MRSA, is commonly used in combination with TMP/SMX or doxycycline. It should not be used alone because of its rapid tendency to select resistant strains [77]. The Sanford Guide recommends the addition of rifampin to TMP/SMX for patients who have an abscess associated with fever, those with large or multiple abscesses, and in severe infections [74]. The only supporting data are from a retrospective study of CA-MRSA SSTIs, in which clinical resolution was achieved in all of six patients treated with a combination of TMP/SMX and rifampin, but in only 6 of 12 patients treated with double-strength TMP/SMX [78]. Rifampin has numerous drug-drug interactions and an unpleasant side-effect profile (eg, discoloration of bodily fluids). In combination with another agent, it introduces complexity and confusion regarding dosing regimens, which in turn may translate into noncompliance. A potential role of rifampin, because of its greater penetration into mucosal tissue, may lie with its ability to eradicate nasal MRSA colonization and potentially reduce the rate of recurrence, but this has not been demonstrated in the setting of CA-MRSA skin infections [79,80].

The activity of clindamycin against CA-MRSA is geographically variable, with a higher prevalence of resistance compared with TMP/SMX. However, compared with TMP/SMX, it has superior activity against *S. pyogenes* and some anaerobes (eg, *Peptostreptococcus*), and has the capability of inhibiting toxin production [81]. Some strains of MRSA display inducible clindamycin resistance. Pretherapy, these strains demonstrate in vitro erythromycin-resistant and clindamycin-sensitive susceptibility patterns. However, when exposed to clindamycin, they develop in vitro resistance to clindamycin. This trait can be detected by the double-disk diffusion assay (D test). The prevalence of such strains is geographically variable and the clinical significance is not well understood, as both clinical cure and treatment failures have been reported [82–87]. In a small retrospective study of invasive CA-MRSA infections in children, clindamycin demonstrated clinical efficacy in patients infected with clindamycin-susceptible CA-MRSA isolates [88]. However, because of lack of published experience, clindamycin is not advocated for use as a sole agent in severe infections [89].

Extended-spectrum tetracyclines, such as doxycycline and minocycline, are also reasonable choices for oral agents against CA-MRSA if local isolates display a high susceptibility rate [90,91]. Minocycline may have a slight advantage over doxycycline in its staphylococcal (MSSA) and streptococcal activity [74]. These drugs should be avoided in children under 9 years old, pregnant patients, and nursing mothers.

Vancomycin is the most commonly used intravenous agent for the treatment of MRSA infections. Although vancomycin has been used for many decades without many alternatives, its poor tissue penetration, increasing staphylococcal MICs associated with clinical failure, and inferior clinical efficacy, compared with antistaphylococcal β-lactams in the treatment of MSSA infections, has raised concerns regarding its efficacy relative to newer agents [92–94]. Alternate intravenous agents with FDA approval for the treatment of MRSA SSTIs include linezolid (Zyvox), daptomycin (Cubicin), and tigecycline (Tygacil). Quinupristin-dalfopristin (Synercid) has in vitro activity against MRSA and an indication for treatment of complicated SSTI; however, it does not currently have specific approval for MRSA infections [66–68].

Linezolid has excellent in vitro activity against MRSA [62], and unlike vancomycin has the ability to suppress toxin production [81]. In a randomized, open-label, multicenter study of complicated SSTIs, based on subgroup analysis, linezolid outcomes were statistically superior to vancomycin at the test-of-cure visit for patients with MRSA infections [63]. However, a reanalysis of this study challenged the differential treatment effect based on the microorganism [95]. Although both daptomycin and tigecycline are FDA-approved for the treatment of complicated SSTIs caused by MRSA, the associated clinical studies are limited by the small number of subjects with documented MRSA SSTIs [96,97].

If indicated, empiric antimicrobial therapy for SSTIs associated with purulence should include agents that have been shown to have adequate in vitro activity against CA-MRSA [12]. The role of CA-MRSA in nonpurulent SSTIs (eg, nonpurulent cellulitis) is unclear. However, in light of the emergence of CA-MRSA in purulent SSTI and the prominent role of MSSA in previous studies of cellulitis, empiric CA-MRSA coverage is recommended. Because streptococci have been shown to be another common cause of cellulitis [25–28,53], it is reasonable to include an agent or agents with in vitro activity against CA-MRSA and *S. pyogenes.*

It should be noted that the clinical efficacy of TMP/SMX for SSTIs caused by Group A streptococci is unclear. In addition, the activity of TMP/SMX is not routinely tested against *S. pyogenes*, and as a result, current resistance rates of *S. pyogenes* to TMP/SMX are unknown. Although there is evidence that TMP/SMX has in vitro activity [98,99] and some clinical efficacy in infections caused by *S. pyogenes* [100,101], the most recent Centers for Disease Control and Prevention guidelines do not advocaté use of this agent as monotherapy for patients presenting with cellulitis [24].

Empiric antimicrobial therapy for infected dog and cat bite wounds should include coverage against *Pasteurella*, streptococci, staphylococci, and anaerobic species [5]. For infected human bites, empiric antimicrobial therapy should include coverage against *Eikenella*, streptococci, staphylococci, and anaerobic species [6]. *S. aureus* has been found in 4%, 20%, and 30% of cat, dog, and human bite infections, respectively, and none were MRSA [5,6]. Although these studies were done before the emergency of CA-MRSA, at the present time colonization rates in human beings remain low, so empiric CA-MRSA coverage is not recommended in these types of infections [102].

Because of inadequate activity against *Pasteurella* or *Eikenella* species, monotherapy with first-generation cephalosporins, dicloxacillin, erythromycin, clindamycin, and metronidazole should be avoided [103]. The combination therapy of penicillin plus a cephalosporin has been advocated for the initial treatment of human bites [51]. However, this combination, especially if a first-generation cephalosporin is used, does not cover β-lactamase producing anaerobes [6]. Empirical regimens for marine- and freshwater-acquired infection, should cover *Vibrio* and *Aeromonas* species, respectively, with agents such as third-generation cephalosporins (eg, cefotaxime) and fluoroquinolones.

The management of necrotizing SSTI in the ED involves aggressive resuscitation, hemodynamic stabilization, initiation of antibiotics, and surgical consultation. Broad-spectrum empiric antimicrobial therapy should be initiated as soon as possible once the diagnosis is suspected. The spectrum of antibiotic coverage should include gram-positive, gram-negative, and anaerobic organisms, with special attention to resistant organisms (eg, CA-MRSA) [13]. Suitable multidrug regimens include vancomycin plus piperacillin or tazobactam plus clindamycin. Clindamycin have been shown to inhibit toxin production with streptococcal and clostridial infections [104–106], which in turn may be an important intervention in controlling the inflammatory response. One observational study of children with invasive streptococcal infections found superior clinical outcomes in patients receiving antibiotics inhibiting protein synthesis, compared with agents active at the cell wall [107]. In a more recent study, clindamycin and linezolid, both protein synthesis inhibitors at the ribosomal level, were shown to have the capability to suppress toxin production in CA-MRSA strains [81].

The optimal duration of antimicrobial therapy of SSTI is unknown and is ultimately dependent on how the infection responds. Most SSTIs are treated with a 7 to 10 day course of antimicrobial therapy. A shorter course of 3 to 5 days may be appropriate for infections associated with a drainable abscess, though this recommendation is not based on any comparative studies. Complicated cases, such as infections associated with osteomyelitis, an immunocompromising condition, or diminished vascular supply may require a longer duration of therapy. In a randomized, double-blind, placebo-controlled trial of 87 subjects with uncomplicated cellulitis, there was no significant difference in clinical outcome at 14 and 28 days of therapy among subjects who were treated with 5 days, compared with 10 days, of antimicrobial therapy [108]. In a recent retrospective cohort study of 492 subjects with CA-MRSA SSTIs, subjects who had a successful outcome received antibiotics for a median duration of 10 days (interquartile range, 7–14 days) [60].

Disposition

The majority of patients with SSTI can be treated as outpatients. Hospitalization is indicated for patients with hemodynamic instability, altered mental status, severe infection (including those requiring formal operative intervention), intractable nausea and vomiting, the presence of immunocompromising infection, failure of outpatient therapy, and poor social support. The latest IDSA SSTI guidelines indicate hospitalization should be considered in patients with "hypotension and/or an elevated creatinine level, low serum bicarbonate level, elevated creatine phosphokinase level (2–3 times the upper limit of normal), marked left shift, or a C-reactive protein level > 13 mg/L" [4].

Studies of risk factors for mortality, complications, and treatment failures in patients with SSTIs exist [109–111]; however, only a few small studies have attempted to determine a set of variables that may predict the need for (and benefit from) hospitalization [112]. In a study of patients with extremity cellulitis, independent predictors of "need" for hospital admission were a history of diabetes, temperature, hand infections, induration, area greater than 70 cm^2, and the absence of fluctuance. The need for hospitalization was defined as hospital stay greater than 24 hours, operative incision and drainage, or failed outpatient management [112].

In an expert panel recommendation on the management of SSTIs [1], the panel classified patients with SSTIs into four classes: Class I was afebrile and healthy, other than cellulitis; Class 2 was febrile and ill-appearing, but with no unstable comorbidies; Class III was toxic appearing, or with at least one unstable comorbidity or a limb-threatening infection; and Class IV was with a sepsis syndrome or life-threatening infection (eg, necrotizing fasciitis).

For Class I patients, outpatient care on oral antimicrobials was recommended. For the Class IV patients, hospital admission was recommended. For both the Class II and Class III patients, a period of observation, and depending on the outcome, either outpatient care on oral or intravenous (home or infusion center delivered) antimicrobials or hospital admission was recommended. The proposed classification system does not address the most important question as to which patients actually achieve benefit from hospitalization. Most EDs do not have observation units. In addition, for most patients and settings, outpatient parenteral antimicrobial therapy is not feasible or practical.

Some EDs may have observation units that are either run by emergency physicians or general internists. SSTIs are among the most common reason for admission to an observation unit [113]. For ED physicians, it is not unusual to encounter patients who initially present with worrisome clinical findings and equivocal criteria for hospital admission, but after a few simple interventions (eg, intravenous fluids, antipyretics) and a period of observation, they become suitable for outpatient therapy. In some instances, if feasible, patients are brought back to the ED for a few additional doses of intravenous antibiotics, or are treated at home with intravenous antimicrobial therapy [114,115].

For the appropriate indication, dalbavancin (administered in two doses, 1 week apart [69]) may provide a potentially attractive alternative and avert hospitalization for otherwise stable patients who are thought to require parenteral antibiotic therapy or for whom noncompliance is a concern.

Infection control

Since the majority of SSTIs presenting to the ED are likely to be caused by CA-MRSA [12], it would be ideal for all these patients to be placed in private rooms with MRSA contact precautions until culture results are available. However, many EDs are currently dealing with severe overcrowding issues, and isolation capacity is extremely limited. Similarly, because of a limited number of isolation beds in the hospitals, such patients often endure long waits for admission, which in turn results in delays in ED patient flow and disposition. Rapid real-time polymerase chain reaction assay for MRSA may allow rapid identification of these patients and in turn better facilitate infection control measures [116].

MRSA isolation precautions that are used in most hospitals were developed in the era of hospital-associated MRSA. Their utility in the era in which CA-MRSA is prevalent in the community at large is unclear. However, it is known that CA-MRSA strains can spread within hospitals [117]. A common scenario in many facilities is that SSTI patients are admitted without MRSA precautions, then placed in isolation 2 days later when MRSA is confirmed. Although this scenario is clearly suboptimal, it may be impractical to admit every SSTI patient to a private room with MRSA precautions. Because it is known that MRSA is now a likely cause of SSTI, a cohorting strategy for admitted SSTI patients may help reduce nosocomial spread [118]. Whether the infection is caused by MRSA or MSSA, standard precautions should be used for any patient with a purulent wound to prevent exposing other patients or personnel to infected material. Gloves should always be used when handling purulent material, such as when performing incision and drainage or changing dressings of infected wounds. Gowns and eye protection should be used for procedures that are likely to generate splashes or sprays of fluids [24]. Frequent handwashing should always be encouraged in the ED.

MRSA decolonization should be considered in patients with recurrent, active MRSA infections not responding to appropriate therapy, or MRSA infection occurring in closely-associated cohorts (eg, MRSA infection in a family) [24]. Although the efficacy of commonly prescribed decolonization regimens in the prevention of recurrent CA-MRSA skin infections has not been studied, commonly prescribed agents for the purpose of decolonization in the United States includes mupirocin 2% nasal ointment plus chlorhexidine 4% skin cleanser. In a randomized controlled trail, treatment with topical mupirocin, chlorhexidine gluconate washes, oral rifampin, and doxycycline for 7 days was safe and effective in eradicating MRSA colonization in hospitalized patients for at least 3 months [80].

Proper decolonization practices require obtaining cultures from multiple body sites (eg, nares, axilla, groin), performing special susceptibility testing (eg, mupirocin) [119], and educating and possibly treating the patient's family or other close contacts [24]. EDs may not be the optimal place to initiate these interventions. However, many patients do not have access to primary care physicians and EDs are the only site for their medical care. Initiating a decolonization regimen, in selected cases, without obtaining cultures or special susceptibility testing and not involving the family is not uncommon. Although this practice may not be the optimal or preferred way, it is often the only opportunity to initiate a potential therapy for patients who have limited amount of resources and poor follow-up capability.

Summary

The most important new development in the area of SSTI is the increased prevalence of CA-MRSA, a phenomenon largely recognized and studied in ED populations. There are no clinical or epidemiologic risk factors that can reliably exclude MRSA. The emergence of CA-MRSA has made a significant impact in the empiric treatment of SSTIs.

The misclassification of a deep abscess as cellulitis is a common pitfall. The presence of an underlying deep abscess should be considered in patients with cellulitis who fail initial antimicrobial therapy. Treatment failure may be caused by an undrained abscess that was missed on the initial presentation, rather than inadequate antimicrobial therapy. Ultrasonography can be useful in the identification of deep abscesses, especially in cases in which the physical examination is equivocal or there is a broad area of what appears to be cellulitis. Wound and blood cultures can be of value in selected patients with SSTIs; however, their routine performance, clinical utility, and cost-effectiveness in all types of SSTIs are debatable.

The recognition of a necrotizing SSTI, especially in the early stages, is extremely difficult. The utility of the LRINEC score is limited in that it needs to be prospectively validated in patients for whom the diagnosis of necrotizing SSTI is not apparent on initial history and physical examination. Protein synthesis inhibitors (eg, clindamycin, linezolid) have a potential role in the management of necrotizing SSTIs. The majority of patients with SSTI can be treated as outpatients. Prospectively derived sets of variables that may predict the need for (and benefit from) hospitalization in patients with SSTIs are insufficient at this time, and further studies in this area are indicated.

References

[1] Eron LJ, Lipsky BA, Low DE, et al. Managing skin and soft tissue infections: expert panel recommendations on key decision points. J Antimicrob Chemother 2003;52(Suppl 1): i3–17.

[2] DiNubile MJ, Lipsky BA. Complicated infections of skin and skin structures: when the infection is more than skin deep. J Antimicrob Chemother 2004;53(Suppl 2):ii37–50.

[3] Center for Drug Evaluation and Research (CDER). Uncomplicated and complicated skin and skin structure infections: developing antimicrobial drugs for treatment. Guidance for industry. Available at: http://www.fda.gov/cder/guidance/2566dft.pdf. Accessed November 20, 2007.

[4] Stevens DL, Bisno AL, Chambers HF, et al. Practice guidelines for the diagnosis and management of skin and soft-tissue infections. Clin Infect Dis 2005;41(10):1373–406.

[5] Talan DA, Citron DM, Abrahamian FM, et al. Bacteriologic analysis of infected dog and cat bites. N Engl J Med 1999;340(2):85–92.

[6] Talan DA, Abrahamian FM, Moran GJ, et al. Clinical presentation and bacteriologic analysis of infected human bites in patients presenting to emergency departments. Clin Infect Dis 2003;37(11):1481–9.

[7] Moet GJ, Jones RN, Biedenbach DJ, et al. Contemporary causes of skin and soft tissue infections in North America, Latin America, and Europe: report from the SENTRY

Antimicrobial Surveillance Program (1998–2004). Diagn Microbiol Infect Dis 2007;57(1): 7–13.

[8] Rennie RP, Lones RN, Mutnick AH, et al. Occurrence and antimicrobial susceptibility patterns of pathogens isolated from skin and soft tissue infections: report from the SENTRY Antimicrobial Surveillance Program (United States and Canada, 2000). Diagn Microbiol Infect Dis 2003;45(4):287–93.

[9] Klevens RM, Morrison MA, Nadle J, et al. Invasive methicillin-resistant *Staphylococcus aureus* infections in the United States. J Am Med Assoc 2007;298(15):1763–71.

[10] Frazee BW, Lynn J, Charlebois ED, et al. High prevalence of methicillin-resistant *Staphylococcus aureus* in emergency department skin and soft tissue infections. Ann Emerg Med 2005;45(3):311–20.

[11] Moran GJ, Amii RN, Abrahamian FM, et al. Methicillin-resistant *Staphylococcus aureus* in community-acquired skin infections. Emerg Infect Dis 2005;11(6):928–30.

[12] Moran GJ, Krishnadasan A, Gorwitz RJ, et al. Methicillin-resistant *S. aureus* infections among patients in the emergency department. N Engl J Med 2006;355(7):666–74.

[13] Miller LG, Perdreau-Remington F, Rieg G, et al. Necrotizing fasciitis caused by community-associated methicillin-resistant *Staphylococcus aureus* in Los Angeles. N Engl J Med 2005;352(14):1445–53.

[14] Diep BA, Gill SR, Chang RF, et al. Complete genome sequence of USA300, an epidemic clone of community-acquired methicillin-resistant *Staphylococcus aureus*. Lancet 2006; 367(9512):731–9.

[15] Voyich JM, Otto M, Mathema B, et al. Is Panton-Valentine leukocidin the major virulence determinant in community-associated methicillin-resistant *Staphylococcus aureus* disease? J Infect Dis 2006;194(12):1761–70.

[16] Lina G, Piemont Y, Godail-Gamot F, et al. Involvement of Panton-Valentine leukocidin-producing *Staphylococcus aureus* in primary skin infections and pneumonia. Clin Infect Dis 1999;29(5):1128–32.

[17] Vandenesch F, Naimi T, Enright MC, et al. Community-acquired methicillin-resistant *Staphylococcus aureus* carrying Panton-Valentine leukocidin genes: worldwide emergence. Emerg Infect Dis 2003;9(8):978–84.

[18] Gillet Y, Issartel B, Vanhems P, et al. Association between *Staphylococcus aureus* strains carrying gene for Panton-Valentine leukocidin and highly lethal necrotizing pneumonia in young immunocompetent patients. Lancet 2002;359(9308):753–9.

[19] Labandeira-Rey M, Couzon F, Boisset S, et al. *Staphylococcus aureus* Panton-Valentine leukocidin causes necrotizing pneumonia. Science 2007;315(5815):1130–3.

[20] Wang R, Braughton KR, Kretschmer D, et al. Identification of novel cytolytic peptides as key virulence determinants for community-associated MRSA. Nat Med 2007;13(12): 1510–4.

[21] Miller LG, Perdreau-Remington F, Bayer AS, et al. Clinical and epidemiologic characteristics cannot distinguish community-associated methicillin-resistant *Staphylococcus aureus* infection from methicillin-susceptible *S. aureus* infection: a prospective investigation. Clin Infect Dis 2007;44(4):471–82.

[22] Skiest DJ, Brown K, Cooper TW, et al. Prospective comparison of methicillin-susceptible and methicillin-resistant community-associated *Staphylococcus aureus* infections in hospitalized patients. J Infect 2007;54(5):427–34.

[23] Naimi TS, LeDell KH, Como-Sabetti K, et al. Comparison of community- and health care-associated methicillin-resistant *Staphylococcus aureus* infection. J Am Med Assoc 2003;290(22):2976–84.

[24] Gorwitz RJ, Jernigan DB, Powers JH, et al, and Participants in the CDC-Convened Experts' Meeting on Management of MRSA in the Community. Strategies for clinical management of MRSA in the community. Summary of an experts' meeting convened by the Centers for Disease Control and Prevention, 2006. Available at: http://www.cdc.gov/ncidod/dhqp/ar_mrsa_ca.html. Accessed November 20, 2007.

[25] Hook EW, Hooton TM, Horton CA, et al. Microbiologic evaluation of cutaneous cellulitis in adults. Arch Intern Med 1986;146(2):295–7.

[26] Sigurdsson AF, Gudmundsson S. The etiology of bacterial cellulitis as determined by fine-needle aspiration. Scand J Infect Dis 1989;21(5):537–42.

[27] Sachs MK. The optimum use of needle aspiration in the bacteriologic diagnosis of cellulitis in adults. Arch Intern Med 1990;150(9):1907–12.

[28] Duvanel T, Auckenthaler R, Rohner P, et al. Quantitative cultures of biopsy specimens from cutaneous cellulitis. Arch Intern Med 1989;149(2):293–6.

[29] Bernard P, Bedane C, Mounier M, et al. Streptococcal cause of erysipelas and cellulitis in adults. A microbiologic study using a direct immunofluorescence technique. Arch Dermatol 1989;125(6):779–82.

[30] Chartier C, Grosshans E. Erysipelas. Int J Dermatol 1990;29(7):459–67.

[31] Eriksson B, Jorup-Ronstrom C, Karkkonen K, et al. Erysipelas: clinical and bacteriologic spectrum and serological aspects. Clin Infect Dis 1996;23(5):1091–8.

[32] Kielhofner MA, Brown B, Dall L. Influence of underlying disease process on the utility of cellulitis needle aspirates. Arch Intern Med 1988;148(11):2451–2.

[33] Squire BT, Fox JC, Anderson C. ABSCESS: applied bedside sonography for convenient evaluation of superficial soft tissue infections. Acad Emerg Med 2005;12(7):601–6.

[34] Tayal VS, Hasan N, Norton HJ, et al. The effect of soft-tissue ultrasound on the management of cellulitis in the emergency department. Acad Emerg Med 2006;13(4):384–8.

[35] Wong CH, Chang HC, Pasupathy S, et al. Necrotizing fasciitis: clinical presentation, microbiology, and determinants of mortality. J Bone Joint Surg Am 2003;85-A(8):1454–60.

[36] McHenry CR, Piotrowski JJ, Petrinic D, et al. Determinants of mortality for necrotizing soft-tissue infections. Ann Surg 1995;221(5):558–65.

[37] Elhabash S, Lee L, Farrow B, et al. Characteristics and microbiology of patients presenting with necrotizing fasciitis. Presented at the Association of VA Surgeons 31st Annual Meeting. Little Rock: Arkansas; May 10–12, 2007.

[38] Summanen PH, Talan DA, Strong C, et al. Bacteriology of skin and soft-tissue infections: comparison of infections in intravenous drug users and individuals with no history of intravenous drug use. Clin Infect Dis 1995;20(Suppl 2):S279–82.

[39] Anaya DA, Dellinger EP. Necrotizing soft-tissue infection: diagnosis and management. Clin Infect Dis 2007;44(5):705–10.

[40] Elliott DC, Kufera JA, Myers RA. Necrotizing soft tissue infections. Risk factors for mortality and strategies for management. Ann Surg 1996;224(5):672–83.

[41] Green RJ, Dafoe DC, Raffin TA. Necrotizing fasciitis. Chest 1996;110(1):219–29.

[42] Pannaraj PS, Hulten KG, Gonzalez BE, et al. Infective pyomyositis and myositis in children in the era of community-acquired, methicillin-resistant Staphylococcus aureus infection. Clin Infect Dis 2006;43(8):953–60.

[43] Dehority W, Wang E, Vernon PS, et al. Community-associated methicillin-resistant Staphylococcus aureus necrotizing fasciitis in a neonate. Pediatr Infect Dis J 2006;25(11):1080–1.

[44] Wong CH, Tan SH, Kurup A, et al. Recurrent necrotizing fasciitis caused by methicillin-resistant Staphylococcus aureus. Eur J Clin Microbiol Infect Dis 2004;23(12):909–11.

[45] Abrahamian FM, Shroff SD. Use of routine wound cultures to evaluate cutaneous abscesses for community-associated methicillin-resistant Staphylococcus aureus. Ann Emerg Med 2007;50(1):66–7.

[46] Lee MC, Rios AM, Aten MF, et al. Management and outcome of children with skin and soft tissue abscesses caused by community-acquired methicillin-resistant Staphylococcus aureus. Pediatr Infect Dis J 2004;23(2):123–7.

[47] Miller LG, Quan C, Shay A, et al. A prospective investigation of outcomes after hospital discharge for endemic, community-acquired methicillin-resistant and -susceptible Staphylococcus aureus skin infection. Clin Infect Dis 2007;44(4):483–92.

[48] Rajendran PM, Young D, Maurer T, et al. Randomized, double-blind, placebo-controlled trial of cephalexin for treatment of uncomplicated skin abscesses in a population at risk for

community-acquired methicillin-resistant *Staphylococcus aureus* infection. Antimicrobial Agents Chemother 2007;51(11):4044–8.

[49] Perl B, Gottehrer NP, Raveh D, et al. Cost-effectiveness of blood cultures for adult patients with cellulitis. Clin Infect Dis 1999;29(6):1483–8.

[50] Bates DW, Goldman L, Lee TH. Contaminant blood cultures and resource utilization. The true consequences of false-positive results. J Am Med Assoc 1991;265(3):365–9.

[51] Swartz MN. Cellulitis. N Engl J Med 2004;350(9):904–12.

[52] Nguyen HB, Rivers EP, Abrahamian FM, et al. Severe sepsis and septic shock: review of the literature and emergency department management guidelines. Ann Emerg Med 2006;48(1): 28–54.

[53] Newell PM, Norden CW. Value of needle aspiration in bacteriologic diagnosis of cellulitis in adults. J Clin Microbiol 1988;26(3):401–4.

[54] Stamenkovic I, Lew PD. Early recognition of potentially fatal necrotizing fasciitis. The use of frozen-section biopsy. N Engl J Med 1984;310(26):1689–93.

[55] Majeski J, Majeski E. Necrotizing fasciitis: improved survival with early recognition by tissue biopsy and aggressive surgical treatment. South Med J 1997;90(11):1065–8.

[56] Ault MJ, Geiderman J, Sokolov R. Rapid identification of group A streptococcus as the cause of necrotizing fasciitis. Ann Emerg Med 1996;28(2):227–30.

[57] Wong CH, Khin LW, Heng KS, et al. The LRINEC (Laboratory Risk Indicator for Necrotizing Fasciitis) score: a tool for distinguishing necrotizing fasciitis from other soft tissue infections. Crit Care Med 2004;32(7):1535–41.

[58] Fitch MT, Manthey DE, McGinnis HD, et al. Abscess incision and drainage. N Engl J Med 2007;357(19):e20.

[59] Berg JO, Mössner BK, Skov MN, et al. Antibacterial properties of EMLA and lidocaine in wound tissue biopsies for culturing. Wound Repair Regen 2006;14(5):581–5.

[60] Ruhe JJ, Smith N, Bradsher RW, et al. Community-onset methicillin-resistant *Staphylococcus aureus* skin and soft-tissue infections: impact of antimicrobial therapy on outcome. Clin Infect Dis 2007;44(6):777–84.

[61] Fridkin SK, Hageman JC, Morrison M, et al. Methicillin-resistant *Staphylococcus aureus* disease in three communities. N Engl J Med 2005;352(14):1436–44.

[62] Betriu C, Redondo M, Boloix A, et al. Comparative activity of linezolid and other new agents against methicillin-resistant *Staphylococcus aureus* and teicoplanin-intermediate coagulase-negative staphylococci. J Antimicrob Chemother 2001;48(6):911–3.

[63] Weigelt J, Itani K, Stevens D, et al. Linezolid versus vancomycin in treatment of complicated skin and soft tissue infections. Antimicrobial Agents Chemother 2005;49(6):2260–6.

[64] Carpenter CF, Chambers HF. Daptomycin: another novel agent for treating infections due to drug-resistant gram-positive pathogens. Clin Infect Dis 2004;38(7):994–1000.

[65] Stein GE, Craig WA. Tigecycline: a critical analysis. Clin Infect Dis 2006;43(4):518–24.

[66] Jones RN, Ballow CH, Acar J, et al. World-wide evaluation of quinupristin-dalfopristin (Q/D) (Synercid): Antimicrobial activity directed against resistant Gram-positive pathogens: Report from the global SMART study. Presented at the 39th Interscience Conference on Antimicrobial Agents and Chemotherapy, San Francisco, USA, 1999. Abstract 1262. p. 263. American Society for Microbiology, Washington, D.C.

[67] Drew RH, Perfect JR, Srinath L, et al. Treatment of methicillin-resistant *Staphylococcus aureus* infections with quinupristin-dalfopristin in patients intolerant of or failing prior therapy. J Antimicrob Chemother 2000;46(5):775–84.

[68] Nichols RL, Graham DR, Barriere SL, et al. Treatment of hospitalized patients with complicated Gram-positive skin and skin structure infections: two randomized, multicenter studies of quinupristin/dalfopristin versus cefazolin, oxacillin or vancomycin. Synercid Skin and Skin Structure Infection Group. J Antimicrob Chemother 1999;44(2):263–73.

[69] Jauregui LE, Babazadeh S, Seltzer E, et al. Randomized, double-blind comparison of once-weekly dalbavancin versus twice-daily linezolid therapy for the treatment of complicated skin and skin structure infections. Clin Infect Dis 2005;41(10):1407–15.

[70] Saravolatz LD, Pawlak J, Johnson LB. Comparative activity of telavancin against isolates of community-associated methicillin-resistant *Staphylococcus aureus*. J Antimicrob Chemother 2007;60(2):406–9.

[71] Van Bambeke F, Van Laethem Y, Courvalin P, et al. Glycopeptide antibiotics: from conventional molecules to new derivatives. Drugs 2004;64(9):913–36.

[72] Rouse MS, Steckelberg JM, Patel R. In vitro activity of ceftobiprole, daptomycin, linezolid, and vancomycin against methicillin-resistant staphylococci associated with endocarditis and bone and joint infection. Diagn Microbiol Infect Dis 2007;58(3):363–5.

[73] Arpida. Intravenous iclaprim. Available at: http://www.arpida.ch/index.php?MenuID= 13&UserID=1&ContentID=65. Accessed November, 2007.

[74] Gilbert DN, Moellering RC, Eliopoulos GM, et al. The Sanford Guide to antimicrobial therapy. 37th edition. Sperryville (VA): Antimicrobial Therapy, Inc; 2007.

[75] Bruun JN, Ostby N, Bredesen JE, et al. Sulfonamide and trimethoprim concentrations in human serum and skin blister fluid. Antimicrobial Agents Chemother 1981;19(1):82–5.

[76] Nowak A, Kadykow M, Klimowicz A. Penetration of trimethoprim and sulfamethoxazole into skin blister fluid. Eur J Clin Pharmacol 1983;25(6):825–7.

[77] Strausbaugh LJ, Jacobson C, Sewell DL, et al. Antimicrobial therapy for methicillin-resistant *Staphylococcus aureus* colonization in residents and staff of a Veterans Affairs nursing home care unit. Infect Control Hosp Epidemiol 1992;13(3):151–9.

[78] Iyer S, Jones DH. Community-acquired methicillin-resistant *Staphylococcus aureus* skin infection: a retrospective analysis of clinical presentation and treatment of a local outbreak. J Am Acad Dermatol 2004;50(6):854–8.

[79] Yu VL, Goetz A, Wagener M, et al. *Staphylococcus aureus* nasal carriage and infection in patients on hemodialysis. Efficacy of antibiotic prophylaxis. N Engl J Med 1986;315(2):91–6.

[80] Simor AE, Phillips E, McGeer A, et al. Randomized controlled trial of chlorhexidine gluconate for washing, intranasal mupirocin, and rifampin and doxycycline versus no treatment for the eradication of methicillin-resistant *Staphylococcus aureus* colonization. Clin Infect Dis 2007;44(2):178–85.

[81] Stevens DL, Ma Y, Salmi DB, et al. Impact of antibiotics on expression of virulence-associated exotoxin genes in methicillin-sensitive and methicillin-resistant *Staphylococcus aureus*. J Infect Dis 2007;195(2):202–11.

[82] Siberry GK, Tekle T, Carroll K, et al. Failure of clindamycin treatment of methicillin-resistant *Staphylococcus aureus* expressing inducible clindamycin resistance in vitro. Clin Infect Dis 2003;37(9):1257–60.

[83] Lewis JS 2nd, Jorgensen JH. Inducible clindamycin resistance in staphylococci: should clinicians and microbiologists be concerned? Clin Infect Dis 2005;40(2):280–5.

[84] Frank AL, Marcinak JF, Mangat PD, et al. Clindamycin treatment of methicillin-resistant *Staphylococcus aureus* infections in children. Pediatr Infect Dis J 2002;21(6):530–4.

[85] Panagea S, Perry JD, Gould FK. Should clindamycin be used as treatment of patients with infections caused by erythromycin-resistant staphylococci? J Antimicrob Chemother 1999; 44(4):581–2.

[86] Rao GG. Should clindamycin be used in treatment of patients with infections caused by erythromycin-resistant staphylococci? J Antimicrob Chemother 2000;45(5):715–6.

[87] Drinkovic D, Fuller ER, Shore KP, et al. Clindamycin treatment of *Staphylococcus aureus* expressing inducible clindamycin resistance. J Antimicrob Chemother 2001;48(2):315–6.

[88] Martinez-Aguilar G, Hammerman WA, Mason EO, et al. Clindamycin treatment of invasive infections caused by community-acquired, methicillin-resistant and methicillin-susceptible *Staphylococcus aureus* in children. Pediatr Infect Dis J 2003;22(7):593–8.

[89] Daum RS. Skin and soft-tissue infections caused by methicillin-resistant *Staphylococcus aureus*. N Engl J Med 2007;357(4):380–90.

[90] Ruhe JJ, Monson T, Bradsher RW, et al. Use of long-acting tetracyclines for methicillin-resistant *Staphylococcus aureus* infections: case series and review of the literature. Clin Infect Dis 2005;40(10):1429–34.

[91] Ruhe JJ, Menon A. Tetracyclines as an oral treatment option for patients with community onset skin and soft tissue infections caused by methicillin-resistant Staphylococcus aureus. Antimicrobial Agents Chemother 2007;51(9):3298–303.

[92] Deresinski S. Vancomycin and *Staphylococcus aureus*—an antibiotic enters obsolescence. Clin Infect Dis 2007;44(12):1543–8.

[93] Mohr JF, Murray BE. Vancomycin is not obsolete for the treatment of infection caused by methicillin-resistant *Staphylococcus aureus*. Clin Infect Dis 2007;44(12):1536–42.

[94] Kim SH, Kim KH, Kim HB, et al. Outcome of vancomycin treatment in patients with methicillin-susceptible *Staphylococcus aureus* bacteremia. Antimicrobial Agents Chemother 2008;52(1):192–7.

[95] Kalil AC, Puumala S, Stoner J. Is linezolid superior to vancomycin for complicated skin and soft tissue infections due to methicillin-resistant *Staphylococcus aureus*? Antimicrobial Agents Chemother 2006;50(5):1910.

[96] Arbeit RD, Maki D, Tally FP, et al. The safety and efficacy of daptomycin for the treatment of complicated skin and skin-structure infections. Clin Infect Dis 2004;38(12):1673–81.

[97] Ellis-Grosse EJ, Babinchak T, Dartois N, et al. The efficacy and safety of tigecycline in the treatment of skin and skin-structure infections: results of 2 double-blind phase 3 comparison studies with vancomycin-aztreonam. Clin Infect Dis 2005;41(Suppl 5):S341–53.

[98] Eliopoulos GM, Wennersten CB. In vitro activity of trimethoprim alone compared with trimethoprim-sulfamethoxazole and other antimicrobials against bacterial species associated with upper respiratory tract infections. Diagn Microbiol Infect Dis 1997;29(1):33–8.

[99] Bushby SR. Trimethoprim-sulfamethoxazole: in vitro microbiological aspects. J Infect Dis 1973;128(Suppl):442–62.

[100] Trickett PC, Dineen P, Mogabgab W. Clinical experience: respiratory tract. Trimethoprim-sulfamethoxazole versus penicillin G in the treatment of group A beta-hemolytic streptococcal pharyngitis and tonsillitis. J Infect Dis 1973;128(Suppl):693–5.

[101] Quick CA. Comparison of penicillin and trimethoprim-sulfamethoxazole in the treatment of ear, nose and throat infections. Can Med Assoc J 1975;112(13 Spec No):83–6.

[102] Loeffler A, Boag AK, Sung J, et al. Prevalence of methicillin-resistant *Staphylococcus aureus* among staff and pets in a small animal referral hospital in the UK. J Antimicrob Chemother 2005;56(4):692–7.

[103] Abrahamian FM, Goldstein EJC. Bites. In: Gorbach S, Bartlett JG, Blacklow NR, editors. Infectious diseases. 3rd edition. Maryland: Williams & Wilkins; 2004. p. 1440–6.

[104] Stevens DL, Bryant AE, Hackett SP. Antibiotic effects on bacterial viability, toxin production, and host response. Clin Infect Dis 1995;20(Suppl 2):S154–7.

[105] Stevens DL, Maier KA, Mitten JE. Effect of antibiotics on toxin production and viability of *Clostridium perfringens*. Antimicrobial Agents Chemother 1987;31(2):213–8.

[106] Stevens DL, Gibbons AE, Bergstrom R, et al. The Eagle effect revisited: efficacy of clindamycin, erythromycin, and penicillin in the treatment of streptococcal myositis. J Infect Dis 1988;158(1):23–8.

[107] Zimbelman J, Palmer A, Todd J. Improved outcome of clindamycin compared with beta-lactam antibiotic treatment for invasive *Streptococcus pyogenes* infection. Pediatr Infect Dis J 1999;18(12):1096–100.

[108] Hepburn MJ, Dooley DP, Skidmore PJ, et al. Comparison of short-course (5 days) and standard (10 days) treatment for uncomplicated cellulitis. Arch Intern Med 2004;164(15):1669–74.

[109] Carratala J, Roson B, Fernandez-Sabe N, et al. Factors associated with complications and mortality in adult patients hospitalized for infectious cellulitis. Eur J Clin Microbiol Infect Dis 2003;22(3):151–7.

[110] Benfield T, Jensen JS, Nordestgaard BG. Influence of diabetes and hyperglycemia on infectious disease hospitalization and outcome. Diabetologia 2007;50(3):549–54.

[111] Murray HE, Stiell IG, Wells GA. Defining treatment failure in ED patients with cellulitis. Acad Emerg Med 2001;8(5):478.

[112] Diercks DB, Kuppermann N, Derlet RW, et al. Derivation and validation of a model for the need of hospital admission in patients with extremity cellulitis. Acad Emerg Med 2000;7(5):562.

[113] Roberts R. Management of patients with infectious diseases in an emergency department observation unit. Emerg Med Clin North Am 2001;19(1):187–207.

[114] Corwin P, Toop L, McGeoch G, et al. Randomized controlled trial of intravenous antibiotic treatment for cellulitis at home compared with hospital. BMJ 2005;330(7483):129.

[115] Donald M, Marlow N, Swinburn E, et al. Emergency department management of home intravenous antibiotic therapy for cellulitis. Emerg Med J 2005;22(10):715–7.

[116] Huletsky A, Lebel P, Picard FJ, et al. Identification of methicillin-resistant *Staphylococcus aureus* carriage in less than 1 hour during a hospital surveillance program. Clin Infect Dis 2005;40(7):976–81.

[117] Seybold U, Kourbatova EV, Johnson JG, et al. Emergence of community-associated methicillin-resistant *Staphylococcus aureus* USA300 genotype as a major cause of health care-associated blood stream infections. Clin Infect Dis 2006;42(5):647–56.

[118] Siegel JD, Rhinehart E, Jackson M, et al. Management of Multidrug-Resistant Organisms in Healthcare Settings, 2006. Available at: www.cdc.gov/ncidod/dhqp/pdf/ar/mdroGuideline2006.pdf. Accessed November 20, 2007.

[119] Jones JC, Rogers TJ, Brookmeyer P, et al. Mupirocin resistance in patients colonized with methicillin-resistant *Staphylococcus aureus* in a surgical intensive care unit. Clin Infect Dis 2007;45(5):541–7.

ELSEVIER
SAUNDERS

INFECTIOUS
DISEASE CLINICS
OF NORTH AMERICA

Infect Dis Clin N Am 22 (2008) 117–143

Antimicrobial Prophylaxis for Wounds and Procedures in the Emergency Department

Gregory J. Moran, MD, FACEP, FAAEM[a,b,c,*],
David A. Talan, MD, FACEP, FAAEM, FIDSA[a,b,c],
Fredrick M. Abrahamian, DO, FACEP[a,b]

[a]David Geffen School of Medicine at University of California Los Angeles,
Los Angeles, CA, USA
[b]Department of Emergency Medicine, Olive View–University of California Los Angeles
Medical Center, Sylmar, USA
[c]Department of Medicine, Division of Infectious Disease, Olive View–University of California
Los Angeles Medical Center, Sylmar, CA, USA

Infectious disease specialists are usually in the position of treating an infection that has already occurred. Occasionally, an opportunity arises to intervene before infection takes place. An infection cannot always be predicted before it occurs, but certain circumstances are associated with a higher risk of infection, which presents an opportunity for prophylaxis.

Infectious disease specialists are experienced in antibiotic prophylaxis for certain high-risk groups such as HIV-infected individuals, neutropenic patients, and patients who are immunosuppressed because of therapy for transplant or rheumatologic disease; however, they are seldom confronted with situations in which people with healthy immune systems may benefit from a defined period of antibiotic prophylaxis.

Emergency physicians are often confronted with these situations. Patients frequently present with high-risk traumatic wounds or infectious exposures. Patients also frequently undergo invasive procedures that carry a risk of infection or may cause bacteremia, potentially putting certain patients at risk for endocarditis. Although most traumatic wounds do not require antibiotic prophylaxis, one should recognize those cases in which the risk of infection is high enough to justify prophylaxis.

---

* Corresponding author. Department of Emergency Medicine, Olive View–UCLA Medical Center, 14445 Olive View Drive, North Annex, Sylmar, CA 91342-1438.
E-mail address: gmoran@ucla.edu (G.J. Moran).

0891-5520/08/$ - see front matter © 2008 Elsevier Inc. All rights reserved.
doi:10.1016/j.idc.2007.12.002   *id.theclinics.com*

This article does not discuss exposure to blood and body fluids (eg, occupational needle sticks). Information on post-exposure prophylaxis for needle sticks or other body fluid exposures can be found elsewhere [1–3]. Topics herein include antimicrobial wound infection prophylaxis for high-risk traumatic wounds, including the prevention of rabies and tetanus. This discussion also addresses prophylaxis for infections related to invasive procedures in the emergency department (ED).

Traumatic wounds

Although virtually all wounds are contaminated with bacteria to some extent, only a small fraction will develop an infectious complication. Estimates of the incidence of traumatic wound infection vary tremendously depending on the method of study and the population examined, but most studies have found an incidence of 4.5% to 6.3% [4–7]. The best way to prevent wound infection is thorough wound cleansing and appropriate closure technique. Radiographic imaging and ultrasound can be useful to evaluate for possible foreign bodies [8]. Despite good wound care, some infections will still occur. Antibiotics have an important role in the management of wound infections and a role in the prophylaxis of certain high-risk wounds. Unlike true prophylaxis of a sterile wound before it becomes contaminated (eg, prior to colectomy), prophylaxis in these circumstances is expectant therapy to prevent the development of wound infection in a contaminated but not yet clinically infected wound. Based on the principles of presurgical prophylaxis, if prophylaxis is to be given, antibiotics should be administered in the ED as soon as possible. Typical sterile site surgery prophylaxis is achieved with one dose, whereas treatment of an established wound infection is usually given for 7 to 10 days; for expectant therapy of contaminated wounds, an intermediate duration of 3 to 5 days is recommended.

Much has been written about the "golden period" after injury in which a wound can be safely closed, and opinions differ as to when the increased risk of infection becomes significant. Although some studies have found that delayed closure does seem be associated with an increased infection rate [7], several studies have found that delayed closure does not seem to be a significant factor, at least up to 18 hours after injury [9–12]. Wounds at a low risk of infection (eg, clean facial or scalp wound) can be safely closed up to 24 hours or more. Primary closure is not advised for high-risk wounds (eg, a foot wound in a diabetic patient) if there is a delay of more than several hours.

For the highest risk wounds, in addition to antibiotic prophylaxis, delayed primary closure should also be considered. The risk of wound infection decreases after 4 days of open wound management [13]. Following initial debridement, the wound is covered with a clean dressing, and the patient returns in 3 to 5 days for closure. The wound edges can be trimmed at that time if necessary.

Regardless of whether patients are given prophylactic antibiotics, they should receive good discharge instructions, including a warning that all wounds have some potential for infection. Patients should be instructed in proper wound care and told to return for evaluation if they experience signs of infection such as increasing redness, swelling, pain, or pus. If there is concern for the presence of a foreign body, because of the limitations of wound exploration and imaging tests, patients should be advised of the continued possibility of retained material, especially if associated with the persistence or development of new local symptoms.

Topical antibiotics

Although topical antibiotics such as mupirocin can successfully treat minor wound infections [14] or eliminate colonization [15], the primary use of topical antibiotics in the ED is for prevention of infection in fresh wounds. Topical ointments containing bacitracin, neomycin, or polymyxin are routinely used by many physicians for fresh wounds; a survey of emergency physicians in the United States found that 71% use a topical antibiotic on simple lacerations [16]. Despite the frequent use of topical antibiotics, surprisingly few studies have assessed the efficacy of topical antibiotics after suture closure. Animal studies have shown that topical antimicrobials inside the wound prior to closure may reduce the infection rate in contaminated wounds [17]. One double-blind, randomized human trial found a 5% infection rate with antibiotic ointment compared with an unexpectedly high 17.6% rate with petrolatum control [18]. Other studies have found no significant reduction in infection rates with topical antibiotics [19]. Because of the higher risk of infection with crush injuries when compared with sharp lacerations, some experts recommend topical antibiotics only for stellate wounds with abraded skin edges [20], but this is not based on comparative trial data.

Systemic antibiotics

Although it is tempting to give prophylactic antibiotics to prevent wound infections, there are limitations associated with this strategy. In many situations, prophylactic antibiotics will not reduce the overall rate of infection but may skew the bacteriology toward more unusual or resistant pathogens. To date, no randomized trials have demonstrated a benefit of antibiotic prophylaxis for simple wounds in immunocompetent patients [5,7,10,11,21]. A meta-analysis of randomized trials also supports the lack of benefit for simple wounds [22]. Despite these data, it is still unclear whether a subset of high-risk wounds or patients may benefit from prophylactic antibiotics.

High-risk traumatic wounds

Although it is known that certain types of wounds are more likely to develop infection, studies of prophylaxis for uninfected high-risk wounds are few and generally underpowered. Nevertheless, many experts recommend prophylaxis for some high-risk wounds [23]. Situations in which prophylaxis is sometimes recommended include an immunosuppressed host, high-risk anatomic site, devitalized tissue, wound contamination, and delayed presentation. Open fractures or wounds into joint spaces typically require debridement and irrigation in the operating room. Studies have demonstrated that prophylactic antibiotics reduce the infection rate of wounds associated with open fractures [24,25].

Prospective outcome studies have found an increased infection rate in patients with immune impairment [26–29] Diabetes, malnutrition, renal failure, HIV infection, chemotherapy and steroid treatment, extremes of age, and obesity have been associated with more infectious complications. Patients with cardiac lesions at high risk for endocarditis should receive prophylactic antibiotics as recommended by the American Heart Association (AHA) when undergoing procedures that may induce transient bacteremia, such as the incision and drainage of a large abscess [30]; however, repair of a wound that is not grossly contaminated or infected does not require antibiotic prophylaxis in these patients.

The anatomic site of the wound may influence the risk of infection. Foot wounds become infected more often than those involving other parts of the body, whereas injuries to the head and neck have the lowest rates of complication [7,12,31]. Differences in regional blood flow and the degree of contamination (from environmental sources and endogenous flora) may explain this observation. A small, double-blind, placebo-controlled trial of prophylactic penicillin for intraoral wounds found a trend toward possible benefit, most notably in patients who had through-and-through lacerations [32]. Although hand wounds are often classified as high risk, studies have failed to demonstrate a benefit of antibiotic prophylaxis for simple non-bite hand wounds [9,33–35]. Although the authors are not aware of randomized studies of wounds in which tendons have been lacerated or exposed, antimicrobial prophylaxis for these high-risk injuries is recommended. Prospective studies have not been done to validate antibiotic prophylaxis for a wound involving the relatively avascular cartilage of the ear or nose, but this therapy is recommended.

It is unclear whether the wound mechanism influences the infection rate. Although some studies have found that crush injuries are at higher risk [36], presumably because of the presence of devitalized tissue which is impaired in its ability to resist bacterial growth, other prospective studies suggest that sharp and blunt mechanisms have similar rates of infection [12,31]. The presence of collected blood within a wound acts as a growth medium and has been shown to increase the risk of infection [37]. Wounds contaminated with greater than 10^5 organisms per gram of tissue are at greater risk of infection, although no practical means exist to make this determination at the time of repair [38]. Antibiotic prophylaxis is recommended for wounds that are grossly contaminated and cannot be adequately cleaned. One of the most important local factors promoting infection is the presence of foreign bodies, particularly organic material such as dirt and wood; glass and metal tend to be inert. Other foreign bodies that appear to promote infection are pieces of clothing and shoes (eg, a nail though a tennis shoe) and sutures [39,40]. Soft tissue gunshot wounds appear to be at low risk for infection and do not require antibiotic prophylaxis [41].

Although the available literature does not support the routine use of pro-phylactic antibiotics in simple wounds, and prophylaxis is poorly studied in high-risk subsets, prophylaxis is recommended in select high-risk situations. It is impossible to make generic recommendations that can account for the multiple factors present in any individual patient; therefore, physicians must use their own judgment. Antibiotic prophylaxis is recommended in the fol-lowing high-risk wound situations, especially if multiple factors are present:

- Patients with significant immunocompromise (eg, poorly controlled diabetes, peripheral vascular disease, steroid use, lymphedema, AIDS)
- Open fractures or wounds into joints
- Wounds involving tendons or cartilage
- Wounds that are grossly contaminated and cannot be adequately cleaned, especially if there may be a retained foreign body
- Puncture wounds and crush injuries
- Bite wounds
- Oral wounds
- Wounds with a significant delay (>18 hours) before presentation

The specific antibiotics used for prophylaxis are similar to those used for the treatment of established infections. In most settings, a first-generation cephalosporin, anti-staphylococcal penicillin (eg, dicloxacillin), or macrolide would be appropriate. Penicillin would be an appropriate choice for intrao-ral wounds because of the activity against most common oral pathogens. Amoxicillin-clavulanate is the preferred prophylactic agent for high-risk bite wounds and for grossly contaminated, devitalized wounds in immuno-compromised patients. Although a parenteral dose of antibiotics at the time of repair will more quickly achieve tissue levels, parenteral antibiotics have not been shown to be any more effective than oral antibiotics for wound infection prophylaxis [22].

Although community-associated methicillin-resistant *Staphylococcus au-reus* (CA-MRSA) has emerged as the most common cause of skin infections [42], it is not necessary to include activity against CA-MRSA for most wound prophylaxis. The antimicrobial spectrum of prophylactic antibiotics should be selected based on the bacterial flora that are likely to exist on the skin at the time of injury and other bacteria that may be introduced through wound contamination (eg, bite wounds, marine exposure, barnyard injuries). Currently, carriage rates for MRSA among the general population remain low, and the authors are aware of no studies supporting the use of antibiotic prophylaxis for wounds directed against this pathogen [43]. Nevertheless, prophylactic regimens with activity against CA-MRSA would be logical for patients at high risk for CA-MRSA colonization, such as those with a history of prior CA-MRSA infection or with a close household contact.

Open fracture

Open fracture is considered an emergency because of the risk of subsequent osteomyelitis. Any break in the skin over a fracture that could allow bacteria access to bone should be considered an open fracture. This situation is obvious when bone is exposed or protruding from the wound, but it is still important to consider open fracture for more subtle cases. The position of the soft tissue wound relative to the fracture may be different at the time of examination than at the time of injury, and bacterial contamination of bone may have occurred even if the bone cannot be directly visualized through the wound. Any wound near a fracture should be carefully explored to assess for possible open fracture. If a wound is in close proximity to a fracture, it is should be considered an open fracture. Management of open fractures requires urgent orthopedic consultation because most will need irrigation and debridement in the operating room. Minor open fractures of distal digits appear to have a low risk of infection [44,45], but prophylaxis is recommended for higher risk situations, such as diabetic patients or contaminated wounds.

The use of prophylactic antibiotics to prevent infection resulting from an open fracture goes back to the earliest days of antimicrobials. In 1939, Jensen and coworkers reported that topical sulfanilamide reduced the infection rate in patients with open fracture [46]. Although administration of parenteral antibiotics as soon as possible after injury has become the standard of care for patients with an open fracture, the studies that are the basis for this practice have limitations. Recommendations are based on a small number of studies that generally are more than 30 years old and suffer from a variety of methodologic problems, including co-mingling of prospective and retrospective data sets, inappropriate statistical analysis, and a lack of blinding or randomization [47]. Nonetheless, the data support the conclusion that a short course of first-generation cephalosporins begun as soon as possible after injury significantly lowers the risk of infection when used in combination with good wound management. There is insufficient evidence to support other common management practices, such as prolonged courses or repeated short courses of antibiotics, the use of antibiotic coverage extending to gram-negative bacilli or clostridial species, or the use of local antibiotic therapies such as beads [47]. A Cochrane Database review of 913 participants in seven studies concluded that antibiotics reduce the incidence of early infections in open fractures of the limbs [48]. The use of antibiotics reduced the incidence of early infection when compared with no antibiotics or placebo with a relative risk of 0.41 (95% CI, 0.27–0.63), absolute risk reduction of 0.08 (95% CI, 0.04–0.12), and number needed to treat of 13 (95% CI, 8–25).

Intravenous antibiotics should be administered in the ED as soon as possible to reduce the risk of subsequent osteomyelitis. Cultures of open fractures at the time of initial treatment do not appear to be helpful [49]. The best predictors of infection are the severity of the fracture and the amount of overlying soft tissue damage [50]. Open fractures are divided into different types with progressively greater risk of infection [24]: type 1, an open fracture with a less than 1 cm clean laceration and minimal soft tissue damage; type 2, an open fracture with a 1 cm or greater clean laceration without extensive soft tissue injury, flaps, or avulsion; and type 3, a fracture with extensive soft tissue damage. The Eastern Surgical Society for the Surgery of Trauma has developed treatment guidelines [51]. Antibiotic therapy directed against gram-positive bacteria (eg, a first-generation cephalosporin such as cefazolin) should be administered within 6 hours following type 1 and 2 fractures. The duration of antibiotic therapy should be 24 hours after wound closure. Antibiotic therapy directed against gram-positive and gram-negative bacteria (eg, cefazolin plus an aminoglycoside) should be given within 6 hours following type 3 fractures. Antibiotic therapy should be continued for 72 hours or for 24 hours after wound closure.

Penetrating abdominal wounds

Penetrating abdominal wounds pose a high infection risk because of spillage of intestinal contents into the peritoneum. Antimicrobial agents have been used to prevent infection related to penetrating abdominal injury for many decades. Early uncontrolled studies suggested that the timing of antibiotic administration could impact the development of injury-related infections in patients with penetrating abdominal injuries. Patients receiving antibiotics before surgery had lower rates of postoperative peritonitis [52]. Antibiotics with activity against both aerobic and anaerobic organisms are associated with greater reduction of postoperative infection when compared with regimens without anaerobic activity [53]. A single-agent regimen using a beta-lactam antibiotic with aerobic gram-negative and anaerobic activity is as effective as combined regimens including an aminoglycoside [54]. Twenty-four hours of therapy appears to be adequate [55,56].

Plantar puncture wounds

Plantar puncture wounds represent a unique challenge because of the high risk for complications such as osteomyelitis, which may occur months following an injury. Controversy remains about the optimal management of these cases, largely due to a lack of good scientific data. One study involved 887 patients with puncture wounds of the feet (mostly children who had stepped on a nail) [57]. Cellulitis developed in 8.4% of patients seen within 24 hours of injury compared with 57% of those who waited more than a day before presentation, although this undoubtedly reflects some selection bias of those who sought care. Osteomyelitis ultimately developed in 16 (1.8%)

of the 887 patients, and *Pseudomonas* was identified in 13. Another study found that infection developed in 51 (2.2%) of 2303 patients with foot puncture wounds and osteomyelitis in one (0.04%) [58]. It is likely that many patients with such wounds never present for care; therefore, some estimates of the infection rate are probably too high. Other reports have confirmed the risk of osteomyelitis, osteochondritis, and septic arthritis [59]. Although several organisms have been reported in post-plantar puncture osteomyelitis, *Pseudomonas* is the most common. *Staphylococcus aureus* is also commonly isolated from septic arthritis or osteochondritis [60]. Appropriate agents for empiric therapy for osteomyelitis after plantar wounds would include ceftazidime, cefepime, or ciprofloxacin. Cellulitis after foot puncture wounds is not associated with pseudomonal infection and can be treated with antistaphylococcal antibiotics.

It is unclear if prophylactic antibiotics are helpful in plantar wounds because no controlled prospective studies have been published, and controversy exists in terms of recommendations [61,62]. One nonrandomized observational study found that antibiotics reduced the risk of wound infection, but there were several potential confounders [63]. It is clear that antibiotics at initial presentation will not always prevent infection. Of the 16 osteomyelitis cases in the previously mentioned study, 5 were treated at initial presentation with "appropriate" antibiotics in addition to thorough cleansing and debridement [57]. Because no benefit of antibiotic prophylaxis was demonstrated in these cases and because serious infections occur in a small percentage of foot puncture wounds, antibiotic treatment can be reserved for those with evidence of infection or open fracture. Radiographs should be obtained in appropriate cases (eg, stepping on a nail) to identify radio-opaque foreign bodies (ie, metal and glass) and to look for obvious fractures and more subtle periosteal disruption. It is especially important that these wounds be closely inspected for foreign bodies, such as a small piece of shoe rubber, and any foreign material removed as well as possible. Patients should be instructed to return immediately for any sign of infection and should be further advised that symptoms of bony infection may not occur until months later. If a clinician chooses to give antibiotic prophylaxis to a patient with a high-risk plantar puncture wound (eg, diabetic with poor circulation), a fluoroquinolone such as ciprofloxacin would be a reasonable choice [64].

Bite wounds

In the United States, animal bites are a common injury seen in EDs [65]. Dog bites can produce a variety of tissue injury patterns, such as avulsions, lacerations, and crush injuries. A dog's bite can penetrate body cavities, puncture the skull, and break bones. Injury type varies by age. Children younger than 4 years are more susceptible to bites to the head and neck. In contrast, over 80% of injuries in patients over the age of 15 years are to the extremities. Approximately 5% to15% of dog bites become infected. The infection rate for bites to the hand is higher than that for other areas [66].

Cats have long, slender, sharper teeth that usually cause puncture wounds. As many as 80% of cat bites become infected. Wounds that appear uncomplicated can extend into deeper structures such as tendons, joints, vessels, or bone.

Human bites are generally high-risk injuries for infection. The clenched fist injury is the most serious and infection prone. This common injury arises when an individual punches another in the mouth during an altercation, and the teeth penetrate the skin near the metacarpophalangeal joints. The mechanism involves considerable force and can cause injury to deeper structures including fractures, joint penetration, and tendon damage. Infections related to clenched fist injuries can range from a simple cellulitis to severe deep space infection of the hand that requires amputation [67]. Patients presenting with a "fight bite" often present with an established infection rather than immediately after the injury. Infections related to animal and human bites often develop rapidly, within 12 to 24 hours of the injury. The location and type of wound, species of the biting animal, and the medical condition of the patient are factors associated with the probability of developing an infection. Bite wounds tend to have multiple bacteria in high numbers. The bacterial count usually increases dramatically several hours after the injury. Infections are more common in the very young, elderly, and the immunocompromised. Cultures of the uninfected bite wound do not predict which patients will become infected nor do they reveal the subsequently identified pathogens in those who do [68,69].

Proper wound management is critical in preventing infection of bite wounds (and other highly contaminated wounds). The wound should be irrigated with a large amount of saline at high pressure; this irrigation is the most important factor in decreasing the bacterial load. It can be accomplished by using a 12-mL or larger syringe attached to an 18-gauge catheter. All visible foreign material should be removed, and devitalized tissue should be debrided. Approximately 150 to 300 mL or 50 to 100 mL/cm is recommended. Concentrated forms of povidone-iodine, hydrogen peroxide, or ethyl alcohol should not be used as irrigating solutions because they can cause further tissue damage that may impair healing [70].

Primary wound closure and prophylactic antibiotics are the two most controversial issues in dealing with bite wounds. Although multiple small studies have evaluated the utility of primary closure in bite wounds, unfortunately, no reliable prospective data exist to support standardized guidelines on primary closure [71]. These studies do support the practice of primary closure in selected wounds after careful wound preparation. Facial wounds have a lower overall risk of infection than wounds in other locations, and a cosmetic result is more critical. Primary closure is not appropriate for most puncture wounds or wounds that are both open lacerations and punctures. Primary closure should be considered only in special circumstances for other high-risk wounds such as those involving the hand.

The decision about primary closure of bite wounds should be based on a risk-benefit analysis of the characteristics of the individual wound. Potential advantages of primary closure include less need for repeat visits, a better cosmetic result, and protection of underlying structures. Wounds that heal by secondary intention tend to undergo more scarring and contraction than those that are approximated with sutures. In addition, for some areas such as the scalp or pretibial area, the surrounding skin is sometimes unable to completely close the defect. Exposed tendons, vessels, and bone can desiccate in an open wound. The main disadvantage is that primary closure of contaminated wounds can increase the risk of infection. Because of the recognized risk of complications related to bite wounds, it is prudent to document a discussion with the patient about the potential risks and benefits of wound closure.

Some simple clean wounds can be closed after careful inspection and irrigation. Another option is delayed primary closure, in which the wound is irrigated and debrided, left open, and then re-evaluated 3 to 5 days later for suturing. Closure at that time is possible if the wound remains clean and uninfected. Wound edges may sometimes need to be sharply debrided. Delayed primary closure may give a better cosmetic result than closure by secondary intention.

The role of antibiotic prophylaxis for bite wounds is controversial [22,72]. Prophylactic antibiotics are recommended for patients who have higher risk wounds such as deep punctures or hand injuries and for wounds that are closed primarily. Cat and human bites tend to be associated with more infections than dog bites. The benefit of prophylaxis for lower risk wounds is less clear.

Appropriate antimicrobial prophylaxis for bite wounds must take into the account the bacteriology of these infections. Unlike typical wound infections in which the pathogen is usually Group A streptococcus or *Staphylococcus aureus*, bite wounds tend to have a more complex microbiology derived from the oral flora of the biting animal. These infections tend to be polymicrobial with various streptococci, *Staphylococcus* sp, gram-negative species, and oral anaerobes. One large series of animal bite wound infections reported an average of five isolates per wound [73]. *Pasteurella* sp are the most common, occurring in 50% of dog bite infections and as many as 75% of cat bite infections. Most infections also involve streptococci and staphylococci, and anaerobes including *Fusobacterium*, *Bacteroides*, *Porphyromonas*, and *Prevotella* sp.

Human bite infections also tend to be polymicrobial [74]. *Streptococcus anginosus* is the most common pathogen, found in 52% of infections, followed by *Staphylococcus aureus* and *Eikenella corrodens*, each in 30%. Oral anaerobes are also often present. Human bites have the potential to spread other pathogens, including hepatitis B, hepatitis C, and HIV

[75–78]. Prophylaxis for hepatitis B or HIV should be considered in circumstances in which the bite source is known or suspected to be infected with these viruses [1].

Pasteurella sp are susceptible to penicillin, ampicillin, second- and third-generation cephalosporins, doxycycline, trimethoprim-sulfamethoxazole, fluoroquinolones, clarithromycin, and azithromycin. *Pasteurella* are resistant to cephalexin, dicloxacillin, erythromycin, and clindamycin. Appropriate choices for prophylaxis of dog or cat bite wounds would include amoxicillin-clavulanate or a combination of penicillin plus cephalexin (Table 1). For patients with a penicillin allergy, moxifloxacin or combination therapy with ciprofloxacin and clindamycin has activity against the likely pathogens [79]. Azithromycin may also be effective for the penicillin-allergic patient but has less activity against anaerobes. Because *Eikenella corrodens* is also resistant to cephalexin, dicloxacillin, and clindamycin, human bite wounds are treated with similar regimens. Coverage for CA-MRSA is not recommended because oral colonization of the human and animal mouth with CA-MRSA is unlikely.

Knowledge of the organisms involved in exotic animal bites is based on anecdotal reports. Many of these reports suggest that other animals have oral flora that includes staphylococci, streptococci, and anerobes, similar to domestic animals. Antimicrobial prophylaxis for bites by other mammals is similar to that for dogs and cats (eg, amoxicillin/clavulanate). Rodents can transmit a variety of diseases, including rat-bite fever. This rare infection, manifested by fever and a rash, is caused by either *Streptobacillus moniliformis* or S*pirillum minus*. Penicillin is the drug of choice for treatment of rat-bite fever, but giving routine prophylaxis is probably unnecessary because rat bites have a low risk of infection. Bites from adult macaque monkeys have been known to transmit the potentially lethal virus *Herpesvirus simiae* ("B virus"). The best way to prevent *Herpesvirus simiae* is by aggressive local wound lavage. In at-risk patients (such as those who were bitten by a sick monkey), acyclovir prophylaxis is recommended [80].

Rabies prophylaxis for bite wounds

The possibility of rabies exposure and the need for rabies post-exposure prophylaxis (RPEP) should be evaluated for any mammalian bite wound

Table 1
Antimicrobial prophylaxis for dog, cat, or human bites

Patient	Regimen
Adult or child with no penicillin allergy	Amoxicillin/clavulanate, 875 mg PO BID (20 mg/kg PO BID for children)
Adult with penicillin allergy	Moxifloxacin, 400 mg PO daily, or ciprofloxacin, 500 mg PO BID + clindamycin, 450 mg PO q6h
Child with penicillin allergy	Clindamycin, 10 mg/kg PO q6h + trimethoprim/ sulfamethoxazole, 5 mg/kg PO q12h

[81]. Although human rabies is rare in the United States, RPEP is still commonly given for animal exposures seen in EDs [82,83]. The real challenge in rational RPEP use is to ensure that all true rabies exposures are treated without unnecessarily treating a large number of very low-risk exposures. In the United States, rabies is most commonly reported in animals such as raccoons, skunks, bats, and foxes. Other animals that can potentially transmit the disease include bobcats, coyotes, and mongooses. Smaller mammals such as squirrels, rabbits, mice, and rats are considered to be at a lower risk for transmitting the disease. If attacked by an infected predator, these animals usually succumb quickly; therefore, they have a very limited chance of spreading rabies. Non-mammalian bites (eg, birds and reptiles) pose no risk of rabies transmission.

Rabies virus is a single-stranded negative polarity RNA virus belonging to the genus *Lyssavirus* of the Rhabdoviridae family [84]. After inoculation, the virus is believed to enter muscle cells and multiplies until the concentration is sufficient to allow infectious units to cross the myoneural junction and enter the nervous system through unmyelinated sensory and motor axon terminals. The virus moves proximally via axons and then is transferred cell-to-cell within the central nervous system. The efficacy of RPEP is believed to result from preventing rabies virus from crossing the myoneural junction. Once clinical signs develop, RPEP is ineffective in preventing death.

The pattern of rabies has changed significantly in the United States over the last several decades. Before 1960, most reports of animal rabies collected through national surveillance were from domestic animals, now more than 90% occur in wildlife [85]. Control of rabies in domestic animal populations and the development of RPEP that is virtually 100% effective have led to a decline in human rabies from more than 100 cases per year at the turn of the twentieth century to the current rate of 0 to 2 cases per year; however, at the same time, wild animal rabies has expanded. A variant of rabies virus maintained by raccoons has spread over the last 30 years in the Eastern United States. There have been no documented human rabies cases in the United States associated with the raccoon rabies virus variant, but the use of and expenditures for RPEP have substantially increased as a result of the expanding epizootic [86]. Although wild animals are much higher risk for transmission of rabies, the vast majority of RPEP use in the United States is for domestic animal exposures [87].

General guidelines for proper administration of RPEP have been published by the Immunization Practices Advisory Committee (ACIP) [88], and many local public health agencies publish guidelines that take into account the local rabies epidemiology. RPEP should be given immediately after exposure to any animal that is known or suspected to be rabid and cannot be observed (Fig. 1). An unprovoked attack by a domestic animal is more likely to indicate that the animal is rabid. Bites inflicted while a person is attempting to feed or handle a healthy animal should generally be

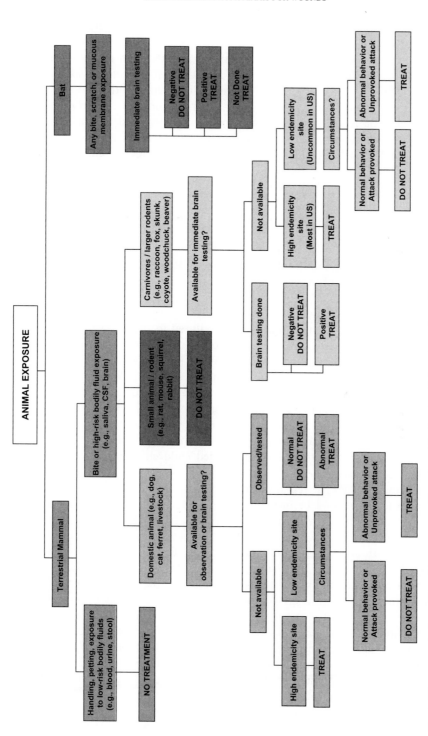

Fig. 1. Management of possible rabies exposure. (*Data from* Abrahamian FM, Talan DA. Rabies postexposure prophylaxis. In: Baren JM, Rothrock SG, Brennan JA, et al, editors. Pediatric emergency medicine. Philadelphia: Elsevier; 2008. p. 754–8.)

considered provoked. A fully vaccinated dog or cat is unlikely to become infected with rabies.

The likelihood that a domestic animal is infected with rabies varies by region. Domestic animal rabies is reported most commonly along the United States–Mexico border and sporadically in areas with enzootic wildlife rabies. In most areas, RPEP is not required for exposure to domestic dogs, cats, or ferrets if the animal appears healthy and is available for 10 days of observation. If the animal is not available for observation, the need for RPEP will depend on the local rabies epidemiology, and local public health officials should be consulted.

Persons with high-risk exposures to animals such as bats, raccoons, skunks, and foxes should be treated immediately unless the geographic area is known to be free of rabies or the animal has already been tested and proven not to be rabid. Persons bitten by domestic animals (eg, dogs or cats) in developing countries are at much higher risk for rabies than in developed countries and should usually receive RPEP. Exposures to animals such as squirrels, rabbits, chipmunks, hamsters, rats, mice, or other rodents almost never require RPEP, but local public health officials should be consulted for regional guidelines.

The majority of human rabies cases acquired in the United States over the last several decades have been due to bat-related virus variants [89]. A bat bite history could be documented in only a few of these cases, suggesting that limited or seemingly insignificant contact with rabid bats may result in transmission of virus. RPEP should now be considered in all situations in which there is a reasonable probability that contact with a bat has occurred, unless prompt laboratory testing of the bat has ruled out rabies infection. Potential contacts include the discovery of a bat in a household area used for sleeping or where there are unattended children or mentally disabled or intoxicated persons.

In almost all RPEP regimens, both rabies vaccine and rabies immune globulin (RIG) should be included. Rabies vaccine provides active immunity, whereas RIG provides passive immunity to protect the patient while an immune response develops to vaccine. Any wounds should be thoroughly cleansed with soap and water and irrigated. RIG is given in a dose of 20 IU/kg body weight. If possible, the entire dose of RIG should be infiltrated around the wound. If this is not possible (eg, wound on a child's finger), the rest should be given intramuscularly in the deltoid or quadriceps muscle. To avoid antigen-antibody antagonism, RIG and rabies vaccine should not be administered at the same site or by the same syringe. Vaccine is given 1.0 mL intramuscularly in the deltoid area for a total of five doses on days 0, 3, 7, 14, and 28. If the exposed person has been previously vaccinated, two doses of vaccine on days 0 and 3 should be given, and HRIG should not be administered [88].

Common pitfalls in the ED management of possible rabies exposures include the failure to wash wounds thoroughly with soap and water, the failure to consider animal behavior and vaccination status, improper administration of RIG or vaccine, failure to consult public health agencies for recommendations, and failure to arrange follow-up care [90]. In a multicenter study of ED management of 2030 animal exposures, use of RPEP was considered inappropriate in 54 cases (40% of those in which it was given) owing to factors including animal availability for observation and exposure in a low endemicity area. RPEP was considered inappropriately withheld from 119 cases (6.3% of those not receiving RPEP), often because a domestic animal was unavailable for observation or testing [87]. EDs should consider developing local practice guidelines for the management of possible rabies exposures in conjunction with local public health agencies. Emergency physicians should have a low threshold for consulting local public health agencies with questions regarding the care of persons with possible rabies exposure. Posting of the 24-hour telephone number of the local Department of Public Health in the ED is recommended.

Tetanus prophylaxis

Although the global incidence of tetanus is high and continues worldwide to claim thousand of lives annually, it remains a rare disease in the United States and other developed countries [91]. Implementation of large-scale tetanus immunization programs, widespread availability of tetanus toxoid vaccine and human tetanus immune globulin (HTIG), and improved wound care management and childbirth practices have all contributed to the dramatic decline in the incidence of tetanus in developed countries.

Although no active immunization practice is considered 100% effective, tetanus immunization has shown to be one of the most effective immunization practices ever developed [92,93]. Despite its proven efficacy, compliance with immunization protocols for patients seeking medical care is less than adequate. A multicenter study assessing compliance with anti-tetanus immunization protocols in EDs in the United States revealed that physicians provided inadequate prophylaxis to approximately 35% of patients with wounds [94]. Ironically, individuals at the highest risk for tetanus (ie, patients with tetanus-prone wounds lacking a history of primary immunization) had the lowest likelihood of receiving the correct prophylaxis. Tetanus surveillance conducted in the United States by the Centers for Disease Control and Prevention (CDC) for the period from 1998 to 2000 revealed that, for patients with tetanus who sought medical care for their acute injury, only 63% of those eligible received tetanus toxoid for wound prophylaxis as recommended by the ACIP (Table 2) [95].

Tetanus surveillance reports indicate that the populations at highest risk for developing tetanus in the United States are the elderly aged 60 or more years (especially those living in rural areas), persons who are not or inadequately vaccinated, and injection drug users [96]. Serologic surveys similarly

Table 2
Recommendations for tetanus prophylaxis in wound management

History of adsorbed tetanus toxoid (doses)	Clean minor wounds	All other wounds[a]		
	Tdap or Td[b] (0.5 mL IM)	TIG (250 U IM)	Tdap or Td[b] (0.5 mL IM)	TIG (250 U IM)
Unknown or less than three	Yes	No	Yes	Yes
Three or more	No[c]	No	No[d]	No

Abbreviations: IM, intramuscular; Tdap, tetanus-diphtheria-acellular pertussis vaccine adsorbed formulated for use in adolescents and adults ≤64 years of age (Boostrix approved for use in persons aged 10 to 18 years; Adacel approved for use in persons aged 11 to 64 years); Td, adult diphtheria-tetanus vaccine adsorbed (minimum age, 7 years); TIG, tetanus immunoglobulin.

[a] Such as, but not limited to, wounds contaminated with dirt, feces, soil, or saliva; puncture wounds; avulsions; and wounds resulting from missiles, crushing, burns, or frostbite.

[b] Tdap should be substituted for a single dose of Td in adolescents aged 11 to 18 years and adults ≤64 years of age who have never received Tdap. The preferred tetanus toxoid-containing vaccine for children aged less than 7 years is the pediatric diphtheria and tetanus toxoid and acellular pertussis vaccine (DTaP). Minimum age for DTaP administration is 6 weeks and maximum age 6 years.

[c] Yes, if ≥10 years have elapsed since the last tetanus toxoid-containing vaccine dose.

[d] Yes, if ≥5 years have elapsed since the last tetanus toxoid-containing vaccine dose.

From Centers for Disease Control and Prevention. Preventing tetanus, diphtheria, and pertussis among adults: use of tetanus toxoid, reduced diphtheria toxoid and acellular pertussis vaccine. MMWR 2006;55(RR-17):1–33.

have identified groups at higher risk of developing tetanus, including persons aged 70 years or more, immigrants from outside North America or Western Europe, persons with a history of inadequate immunization, and persons uneducated beyond grade school [94,97,98].

The decision to initiate post-exposure prophylaxis depends on the type and condition of the wound and the patient's vaccination history. Current tetanus prophylaxis guidelines recommended by the ACIP [96] categorize wounds as either clean, minor wounds, or all other wounds. Examples of "all other wounds" include contaminated wounds (eg, with dirt, feces, soil, or saliva), puncture wounds, avulsions, and wounds resulting from missiles, crush injuries, burns, or frostbite. These wounds are at higher risk for harboring *Clostridium tetani* because they have occurred in an environment in which *C tetani* spores are prevalent, or they are the type of tissue injury that provides low oxygen tension conducive for anaerobic conditions allowing *C tetani* spore germination and proliferation. Other examples of high-risk wounds include infected and neurovascularly compromised wounds, including skin infections in intravenous drug users. Clean, uncontaminated, minor superficial wounds are less likely to harbor *C tetani*.

The two important factors to determine about a patient's vaccination history are whether the patient has had a primary immunization series (ie, at least three doses of adsorbed tetanus toxoid) and the elapsed time period since the last vaccination dose. From the review of medical records in a study evaluating physician compliance with tetanus prophylaxis guidelines among ED patients presenting with wounds, only 20% and 64% of cases had documentation of primary immunization history and the time since last tetanus booster, respectively [94].

In clinical practice, most patients do not remember whether they have received their primary immunization series. Current tetanus prophylaxis guidelines recommend considering an individual as not having had any previous tetanus vaccinations if the history of past immunization is unknown or uncertain [96]. Individuals who have served in the military and those who have attended grade school in North America or Western Europe after 1950 most likely have completed a primary immunization series. Groups such as immigrants from outside North America or Western Europe, those who did not attend US elementary schools, and individuals with an education level not beyond grade school are more likely to lack primary immunization. In a study of tetanus seroprotection rates in ED patients in the United States, even among patients with a history of adequate immunization, immigration was associated with a lack of seroprotection (82% versus 98% among nonimmigrants; risk ratio, 10.0; 95% CI, 5.1–19.5) [94].

Another important vaccination history question is the time elapsed from the last tetanus booster. For low-risk tetanus wounds, it is recommended that a patient receive tetanus prophylaxis if 10 or more years have elapsed since the last tetanus toxoid-containing vaccine dose. For a high-risk tetanus wound, tetanus prophylaxis is recommended if 5 or more years have elapsed since the last dose.

Active immunization is provided by the administration of tetanus toxoid. Several tetanus toxoid preparations are available (Table 3). Tdap, which includes immunization against diphtheria and pertussis (with the acellular pertussis vaccine), is preferred to Td for adults who require a tetanus toxoid-containing vaccine as part of wound management and who have not previously received Tdap. For adults previously vaccinated with Tdap, Td should be used if a tetanus toxoid-containing vaccine is indicated for wound care. Td is given as a 0.5-mL intramuscular dose into the deltoid muscle of the upper arm or the anterolateral aspect of the thigh (the preferred site for small children). A history of a neurologic reaction (eg, encephalopathy) or an immediate anaphylactic reaction is a contraindication to further Td vaccinations. Patients who have experienced an Arthus-type hypersensitivity reaction or a temperature greater than 39.4°C (103°F) following a prior dose of tetanus toxoid often have high serum tetanus antitoxin levels due to too frequent booster injections. These individuals should not be given further routine or even emergency booster doses of Td more frequently than every 10 years.

DTaP is indicated for primary and booster vaccination for children aged 6 weeks to 7 years (ie, prior to the seventh birthday). DTaP is preferred over diphtheria and tetanus toxoids and whole-cell pertussis vaccine adsorbed

Table 3
Tetanus toxoid preparations

Preparation (abbreviation)	Route, 0.5 mL	Indication
Diphtheria-tetanus-pertussis vaccine adsorbed (DTP)	IM	Use in children <7 years old; the pertussis component of DTP can be either whole cell (DTwP) or acellular (DTaP). The acellular version is the preferred preparation.
Diphtheria-tetanus vaccine adsorbed (pediatric) (DT)	IM	Use in children <7 years old if pertussis vaccine is contraindicated.
Diphtheria-tetanus vaccine adsorbed (adult) (Td)	IM	Use as the preferred agent for adults and children ≥7 years old.
Tetanus and diphtheria toxoids and acellular pertussis vaccine adsorbed (Tdap)	IM	Tdap should be substituted for a single dose of Td in adolescents aged 11 to 18 years and adults ≤64 years of age. Boostrix is approved for use in persons aged 10 to 18 years. Adacel is approved for use in persons aged 11 to 64 years.
Tetanus toxoid adsorbed (TTA)	IM	Use in patients who have a contraindication to combined antigens. It is the preferred single-agent formulation due to its greater antigenic effects.
Tetanus toxoid fluid (TT)	IM or SC	Use in patients who have a contraindication to combined antigens or those who are hypersensitive to the aluminum adjuvant in the adsorbed toxoid.

Abbreviations: IM, intramuscularly; SC, subcutaneous.
Data from Abrahamian FM. Tetanus: an update on an ancient disease. Infect Dis Clin Pract 2000;9(6):2233.

(DTwP) due to its lower incidence of local and systemic adverse reactions and improved efficacy [99]. It is given as a 0.5-mL intramuscular dose into the anterolateral aspect of the thigh or the deltoid muscle of the upper arm.

Post-exposure prophylaxis with HTIG is recommended for patients with high-risk wounds who have not completed their primary immunization series (ie, a history of less than three doses of adsorbed tetanus toxoid-containing vaccine) or who are unaware of their vaccination history. The dose for post-exposure prophylaxis is 250 U intramuscularly into the deltoid muscle or anterolateral aspect of the upper thigh muscles (preferred site for infants and small children). For small children, the prophylactic dose may be calculated by the body weight (4.0 U/kg); however, it is best to administer the entire contents of the vial (250 U), because, theoretically, the amount of toxin produced by the organism is independent of the patient's body size. The 250 U dose will provide adequate antitoxin levels for approximately 2 to 3 days after administration and for a period lasting at least 4 weeks

[100]. HTIG should not be given intravenously due to an increased risk for an anaphylactic reaction. There are no specific contraindications to HTIG administration. HTIG is categorized as a pregnancy category C drug and, when indicated, can be given to a pregnant patient. No dosage adjustment is necessary in patients with renal impairment.

Immunosuppressed individuals may receive tetanus toxoid, although there is some question as to whether these patients mount an adequate immunologic response to the vaccine. Both Td and Tdap are categorized as pregnancy category C drugs. Due to a lack of safety data, currently, Tdap is not recommended for administration in pregnant patients. There is no evidence that Td is teratogenic, and it is the recommended tetanus toxoid-containing vaccine in pregnant patients. Both Td and Tdap are acceptable for administration during breastfeeding.

Although the concurrent administration of HTIG with tetanus toxoid may result in some period of delay in the induction of active immunity, the CDC's ACIP tetanus prophylaxis guidelines recommend that HTIG and tetanus toxoid be given at the same time for patients with tetanus-prone wounds who are uncertain about their primary immunization history or who have received fewer than three prior tetanus toxoid doses in the past. These injections should not be administered at the same site or given by the same syringe.

Prophylaxis for emergency department procedures

Endocarditis prophylaxis

For the last several decades, physicians and dentists have been giving antimicrobial prophylaxis to patients at higher risk for endocarditis based on guidelines from the AHA. These guidelines were based on the belief that the risk for endocarditis was increased in the period shortly after a procedure that might be expected to cause transient bacteremia. In recent years, the utility of routine endocarditis prophylaxis has been called into question by several studies [101–103]. It is now recognized that endocarditis is far more likely to develop from random episodes of bacteremia related to routine daily activities than from a specific invasive procedure. Antibiotic prophylaxis is believed to rarely prevent cases of endocarditis, and, in many circumstances, the risk of antibiotics likely exceeds the minimal benefit. As a result, the 2007 AHA guidelines have limited prophylaxis recommendations for patients with the highest risk heart lesions, such as prosthetic valves, unrepaired cyanotic congenital heart lesions, repaired lesions with unepithelialized prosthetic materials, and transplants with valvulopathy, and for patients with history of endocarditis [30].

The AHA guidelines focused on antimicrobial prophylaxis for dental procedures and for many years did not address procedures such as incision and drainage that may also be associated with bacteremia [104]. Since 1990, the guidelines have also discussed prophylaxis for procedures involving infected skin, skin structures, or musculoskeletal tissue (eg, drainage of an abscess). Other sources also recommend antibiotic prophylaxis for abscess incision and drainage in patients at greatest risk for endocarditis [105]. Whether significant bacteremia is likely to occur during drainage of a cutaneous abscess is a matter of controversy. Although some studies suggest that bacteremia does occur during abscess drainage [106], a study of 50 patients with abscesses who had blood cultures 2 and 10 minutes after incision and drainage found that none had bacteremia [107]. Although abscesses are often polymicrobial, staphylococci and streptococci are the organisms most likely to cause endocarditis. The AHA guidelines recommend that the regimen contain an agent active against staphylococci and beta-hemolytic streptococci, such as an anti-staphylococcal penicillin or a cephalosporin. Vancomycin or clindamycin can be administered to patients unable to tolerate a beta-lactam or who are known or suspected to have an infection caused by a methicillin-resistant strain of staphylococcus. Because CA-MRSA is now known to cause the majority of skin and soft tissue infections presenting to EDs (especially abscesses) [42], vancomycin is recommended when prophylaxis is indicated for abscess drainage, or clindamycin if local susceptibility rates are acceptable.

Although some other procedures performed in the ED might carry a risk of causing transient bacteremia, the risk is likely small, and antimicrobial prophylaxis is unlikely to have a benefit. Procedures for which antimicrobial prophylaxis is not recommended include Foley catheter placement, endotracheal intubation, vaginal delivery, and local anesthetic injections (including oral injections).

Prosthetic joints and other implanted materials

Implanted prosthetic joints and other orthopedic implants carry some risk of becoming infected hematogenously. The risk from an individual ED procedure seems to be low, and routine prophylaxis for prosthetic joints is not generally recommended for most dental or gastrointestinal procedures [108,109]. The risk of hematogenous joint infection is thought to be increased in the first 2 years after a total joint replacement, in patients with a history of previous prosthetic joint infection, and in certain other patients with rheumatologic disease or immunosuppresion (Box 1). Prophylaxis should be given to patients in these higher risk categories for procedures such as incision and drainage of an abscess. Prophylaxis is not indicated for those who only have orthopedic pins, plates, or screws. Prophylaxis is not recommended for patients with other implanted foreign bodies, such as dialysis catheters, ventriculoperitoneal shunts, cardiac pacemakers, or defibrillators [110].

Antimicrobial prophylaxis is generally not indicated for urologic procedures in patients with prosthetic joints [111]. Placement of a transurethral

---

Box 1. Patients at potential increased risk of hematogenous total joint prosthetic infection

All patients during the first 2 years after prosthetic joint replacement

Immunocompromised/immunosuppressed patients
Inflammatory arthropathies (eg, rheumatoid arthritis, systemic lupus erythematosus)
Drug-induced immunosuppression
Radiation-induced immunosuppression

Patients with comorbidities
Previous prosthetic joint infections
Malnourishment
Hemophilia
HIV infection
Diabetes
Malignancy

(Foley) catheter generally does not require antimicrobial prophylaxis. Transurethral catheter placement in a patient with urinary retention and confirmed or suspected prostatitis could possibly be associated with bacteremia; therefore, antimicrobial prophylaxis in this setting for high-risk patients with a prosthetic joint, artificial valve, or endovascular graft is recommended.

Chest tubes

Tube thoracostomy is performed in the ED for a number of reasons, including blunt or penetrating chest trauma with hemopneumothorax, as well as spontaneous pneumothorax. Chest tubes are sometimes complicated by infection that can result in empyema. The incidence of infection related to tube thoracostomy may be greater for tubes placed in the ED than for those placed by surgeons in the operating room [112].

The evidence for benefit of prophylactic antibiotics with tube thoracostomy is variable. Two meta-analyses have concluded that antibiotics reduce the incidence of empyema with tube thoracostomy [113,114]; however, the criteria for the diagnosis of empyema and the antibiotics used in the different studies varied, perhaps limiting the validity of the conclusion. A more recent multicenter clinical trial found a low incidence of infection after tube thoracostomy that did not appear to be reduced by prophylactic antibiotics [115]. A practice guideline published in 2000 [116] concluded that "There are sufficient data to recommend prophylactic antibiotic use in patients receiving tube thoracostomy after chest trauma. A first-generation cephalosporin should be used for no longer than 24 hours." Studies that included patients with nontraumatic reasons for tube thoracostomy (eg, spontaneous pneumothorax) have not found a benefit of prophylactic antibiotics.

Summary

Although most traumatic wounds do not require antimicrobial prophylaxis, some situations exist in which it may be appropriate. Higher risk wounds include those in patients with significant immunocompromise, puncture wounds and crush injuries, open fractures or joints, wounds involving tendons or cartilage, wounds that are grossly contaminated and cannot be adequately cleaned, higher risk bite and oral wounds, and wounds with a significant delay (>18 hours) before presentation. Prophylaxis for tetanus or rabies should also be administered when appropriate. Although most invasive procedures performed in the ED are associated with a low risk for infection, patients with the highest risk cardiac lesions or prosthetic joints who are undergoing procedures such as incision and drainage of an abscess should undergo prophylaxis.

References

[1] Moran GJ. Emergency department management of blood and body fluid exposures. Ann Emerg Med 2000;35(1):47–62.
[2] Moran GJ. Pharmacologic management of HIV/STD exposure. Emerg Med Clin North Am 2000;18(4):829–42.
[3] Centers for Disease Control and Prevention. Updated U.S. Public Health Service guidelines for the management of occupational exposures to HBV, HCV, and HIV and recommendations for postexposure prophylaxis. MMWR Recomm Rep 2001;50(RR–11):1–42.
[4] Gosnold JK. Infection rate of sutured wounds. Practitioner 1977;218(1306):584–5.
[5] Hutton PA, Jones BM, Law DJ. Depot penicillin as prophylaxis in accidental wounds. Br J Surg 1978;65(8):549–50.
[6] Rutherford WH, Spence R. Infection in wounds sutured in the accident and emergency department. Ann Emerg Med 1980;9(7):350–2.
[7] Thirlby RC, Blair AJ, Thal ER. The value of prophylactic antibiotics for simple lacerations. Surg Gynecol Obstet 1983;156(2):212–6.
[8] Hill R, Conron R, Greissenger P, et al. Ultrasound for the detection of foreign bodies in human tissue. Ann Emerg Med 1997;29(3):353–6.
[9] Roberts AHN, Teddy PJ. A prospective trial of prophylactic antibiotics in hand lacerations. Br J Surg 1977;64(6):394–6.
[10] Day TK. Controlled trial of prophylactic antibiotics in minor wounds requiring suture. Lancet 1975;2(7946):1174–6.
[11] Baker MD, Lanuti M. The management and outcome of lacerations in urban children. Ann Emerg Med 1990;19(9):1001–5.
[12] Berk WA, Osbourne DD, Taylor DD. Evaluation of the "golden period" for wound repair: 204 cases from a third world emergency department. Ann Emerg Med 1988;17(5):496–500.
[13] Hollander JE. Wound closure options. In: Singer AJ, Hollander JE, editors. Lacerations and acute wounds: an evidence-based guide. Philadelphia: F.A. Davis; 2003. p. 56–63.

[14] Kraus SJ, Eron LJ, Bottenfield GW, et al. Mupirocin cream is as effective as oral cephalexin in the treatment of secondarily infected wounds. J Fam Pract 1998;47(6):429–33.

[15] Wertheim HF, Verveer J, Boelens HA, et al. Effect of mupirocin treatment on nasal, pharyngeal, and perineal carriage of *Staphylococcus aureus* in healthy adults. Antimicrob Agents Chemother 2005;49(4):1465–7.

[16] Howell JM, Chisholm CD. Outpatient wound preparation and care: a national survey. Ann Emerg Med 1992;21(8):976–81.

[17] Edlich RF, Smith QT, Edgerton MT. Resistance of the surgical wound to antimicrobial prophylaxis and its mechanisms of development. Am J Surg 1973;126(5):583–91.

[18] Dire DJ, Coppola M, Dwyer DA, et al. Prospective evaluation of topical antibiotics for preventing infections in uncomplicated soft-tissue wounds repaired in the ED. Acad Emerg Med 1995;2(1):4–10.

[19] Caro D, Reynolds KW. An investigation to evaluate a topical antibiotic in the prevention of wound sepsis in a casualty department. Br J Clin Pract 1967;21(12):605–7.

[20] Edlich RF, Sutton ST. Post repair wound care revisited. Acad Emerg Med 1995;2(1): 2–3.

[21] Edlich RF, Kenny JG, Morgan RF, et al. Antimicrobial treatment of minor soft tissue lacerations: a critical review. Emerg Med Clin North Am 1986;4(3):561–80.

[22] Cummings P, Del Beccaro MA. Antibiotics to prevent infection of simple wounds: a meta-analysis of randomized studies. Am J Emerg Med 1995;13(4):396–400.

[23] Moran GJ, House HR. Antibiotics in wound management. In: Singer AJ, Hollander JE, editors. Lacerations and acute wounds: an evidence-based guide. Philadelphia: F.A. Davis; 2003. p. 194–204.

[24] Gustilo RB, Anderson JT. Prevention of infection in the treatment of one thousand and twenty-five open fractures of long bones. J Bone Joint Surg Am 1976;58(4):453–8.

[25] Gustilo RB, Merkow RL, Templeman D. The management of open fractures. J Bone Joint Surg Am 1990;72(2):299–304.

[26] Berk WA, Welch RD, Bock BF. Controversial issues in clinical management of the simple wound. Ann Emerg Med 1992;21(1):72–80.

[27] Singer AJ, Hollander JE, Quinn JV. Evaluation and management of traumatic lacerations. N Engl J Med 1997;337(16):1142–8.

[28] Rodgers KG. The rational use of antimicrobial agents in simple wounds. Emerg Med Clin North Am 1992;10(4):753–66.

[29] Cruse PJE, Foord R. A five year prospective study of 23,649 surgical wounds. Arch Surg 1973;107(2):206–9.

[30] Wilson W, Taubert KA, Gewitz M, et al. Prevention of infective endocarditis: guidelines from the American Heart Association. Circulation 2007;116(15):1736–54 [Epub 2007 Apr 19].

[31] Gravett A, Sterner S, Clinton JE, et al. A trial of povidone-iodine in the prevention of infection in sutured lacerations. Ann Emerg Med 1987;16(2):167–71.

[32] Steele MT, Sainsbury CR, Robinson WA, et al. Prophylactic penicillin for intraoral wounds. Ann Emerg Med 1989;18(8):847–52.

[33] Haughey RE, Lammers RL, Wagner DK. Use of antibiotics in the initial management of soft tissue hand wounds. Ann Emerg Med 1981;10(4):187–92.

[34] Grossman JAI, Adams JP, Kunec J. Prophylactic antibiotics in simple hand lacerations. JAMA 1981;245(10):1055–6.

[35] Moran GJ, Talan DA. Hand infections. Emerg Med Clin North Am 1993;11(3):601–19.

[36] Cardany CR, Rodeheaver GT, Thacker JG, et al. The crush injury: a high risk wound. JACEP 1976;5(12):965–70.

[37] Krizek TJ, Davis JH. The role of the red cell in subcutaneous infection. J Trauma 1965;5: 85–95.

[38] Robson MC, Heggers JP. Bacterial quantification of open wounds. Mil Med 1969;134(1): 19–24.

[39] Elek SD. Experimental staphylococcal infections in the skin of man. Ann N Y Acad Science 1956;65(3):85–90.

[40] Mehta PH, Dunn KA, Bradfield JF, et al. Contaminated wounds: infection rates with subcutaneous sutures. Ann Emerg Med 1996;27(1):43–8.

[41] Ordog GJ, Wasserberger J, Balasubramanium S, et al. Civilian gunshot wounds—outpatient management. J Trauma 1994;36(1):106–11.

[42] Moran GJ, Krishnadasan A, Gorwitz RJ, et al, for The EMERGEncy ID NET Study Group. Methicillin-resistant *S aureus* infections among patients in the emergency department. N Engl J Med 2006;355(7):666–74.

[43] Kuehnert MJ, Kruszon-Moran D, Hill HA, et al. Prevalence of *Staphylococcus aureus* nasal colonization in the United States, 2001–2002. J Infect Dis 2006;193(2):172–9.

[44] Suprock MD, Hood JM, Lubahn JD. Role of antibiotics in open fractures of the finger. J Hand Surg 1990;15(5):761–4.

[45] Zook EG, Guy R, Russell RC. A study of nail bed injuries: causes, treatment, and prognosis. J Hand Surg 1984;9(2):247–52.

[46] Jensen NK, Johnsrud LW, Nelson MC. The local implantation of sulfanilamide in compound fractures. Surgery 1939;6(1):1–12.

[47] Hauser CJ, Adams CA, Eachempati SR. Surgical Infection Society guideline: prophylactic antibiotic use in open fractures. An evidence-based guideline. Surg Infect (Larchmt) 2006; 7(4):379–405.

[48] Gosselin RI, Roberts I, Gillespie WJ. Antibiotics for preventing infection in open limb fractures. Cochrane Database Syst Rev 2004;(1):CD003764.

[49] Lee J. Efficacy of cultures in the management of open fractures. Clin Orthop Relat Res 1997;339:71–5.

[50] Dellinger EP, Miller SD, Wertz MJ, et al. Risk of infection after open fracture of the arm or leg. Arch Surg 1988;123(11):1320–7.

[51] Luchette FA, Bone LB, Born CT, et al. Eastern Association for the Surgery of Trauma (EAST) working group. Practice management guidelines for prophylactic antibiotic use in open fractures 2000. Available at: www.east.org/tpg.html. Accessed November 11, 2007.

[52] Fullen WD, Hunt J, Altemeier WA. Prophylactic antibiotics in penetrating wounds of the abdomen. J Trauma 1972;12(4):282–9.

[53] Thadepalli H, Gorbach SL, Broido PW, et al. Abdominal trauma, anaerobes, and antibiotics. Surg Gynecol Obstet 1973;137(2):270–6.

[54] Hooker KD, DiPiro JT, Wynn JJ. Aminoglycoside combinations versus beta-lactams alone for penetrating abdominal trauma: a meta-analysis. J Trauma 1991;31(8):1155–60.

[55] Fabian TC, Croce MA, Payne LW, et al. Duration of antibiotic therapy for penetrating abdominal trauma: a prospective trial. Surgery 1992;112(4):788–95.

[56] Luchette FA, Borzotta AP, Croce MA, et al. Practice management guidelines for prophylactic antibiotic use in penetrating abdominal trauma: the EAST Practice Management Guidelines Work Group. J Trauma 2000;48(3):508–18.

[57] Fitzgerald RH, Cowan JDE. Puncture wounds of the foot. Orthop Clin North Am 1975; 6(4):965–72.

[58] Houston AN, Roy WA, Faust RA, et al. Tetanus prophylaxis in the treatment of puncture wounds of patients in the deep south. J Trauma 1962;2:439–50.

[59] Patzakis MJ, Wilkins J, Brien WW, et al. Wound site as a predictor of complications following deep nail punctures to the foot. West J Med 1989;150(5):545–7.

[60] Jacobs RF, McCarthy RE, Elser JM. *Pseudomonas* osteochondritis complicating puncture wounds of the foot in children: a 10-year evaluation. J Infect Dis 1989;160(4): 657–61.

[61] Reinherz RP, Hong DT, Tisa LM, et al. Management of puncture wounds in the foot. J Foot Surg 1985;24(4):288–92.

[62] Joseph WS, LeFrock JL. Infections complicating puncture wounds of the foot. J Foot Surg 1987;26(1 Suppl):S30–3.

[63] Pennycook A, Makower R, O'Donnell AM. Puncture wounds of the foot: can infectious complications be avoided? J Royal Soc Med 1994;87(10):581–3.

[64] Raz R, Miron D. Oral ciprofloxacin for treatment of infection following nail puncture wounds of the foot. Clin Infect Dis 1995;21(1):194–5.

[65] Weiss HB, Friedman DI, Coben JH. Incidence of dog bite injuries treated in emergency departments. JAMA 1998;279(1):51–3.

[66] Cummings P. Antibiotics to prevent infection in patients with dog bite wounds: a meta-analysis of randomized trials. Ann Emerg Med 1994;23(3):535–40.

[67] Dellinger EP, Werts MJ, Miller SD, et al. Hand infections: bacteriology and treatment, a prospective study. Arch Surg 1988;123(6):745–50.

[68] Ordog GJ. The bacteriology of dog bite wounds on initial presentation. Ann Emerg Med 1986;15(11):1324–9.

[69] Fleisher GR. The management of bite wounds. N Engl J Med 1999;340(2):138–40.

[70] Hollander JE, Singer AJ. Laceration management. Ann Emerg Med 1999;34(3):356–67.

[71] Chen E, Horing S, Shepherd SM, et al. Primary closure of mammalian bites. Acad Emerg Med 2000;7(2):157–61.

[72] Callaham M. Prophylactic antibiotics in dog bite wounds: nipping at the heels of progress. Ann Emerg Med 1994;23(3):577–9.

[73] Talan DA, Citron DM, Abrahamian FM, et al. Bacteriologic analysis of infected dog and cat bites. New Engl J Med 1999;340(2):85–92.

[74] Talan DA, Abrahamian FM, Moran GJ, et al. Clinical presentation and bacteriologic analysis of infected human bites in patients presenting to emergency departments. Clin Infect Dis 2003;37(11):1481–9.

[75] Dusheiko GM, Smith M, Scheuer PJ. Hepatitis C virus transmitted by human bite. Lancet 1990;336(8713):503–4.

[76] Cancio-Bello TP, de Medina M, Shorey J, et al. An institutional outbreak of hepatitis B related to a human biting carrier. J Infect Dis 1982;146(5):652–6.

[77] Vidmar L, Poljak M, Tomazic J, et al. Transmission of HIV-1 by human bite. Lancet 1996; 347(9017):1762.

[78] Richman KM, Rickman LS. The potential for transmission of human immunodeficiency virus through human bites. J Acquir Immune Defic Syndr 1993;6(4):402–6.

[79] Goldstein EJC, Citron DM, Merrian CV. Linezolid activity compared to those of selected macrolides and other agents against aerobic and anaerobic pathogens isolated from soft tissue bite infections in humans. Antimicrob Agents Chemother 1999;43(6): 1469–74.

[80] Holmes GP, Chapman LE, Stewart J, et al. Guidelines for the prevention and treatment of B-virus infections in exposed persons. Clin Infect Dis 1995;20(2):421–39.

[81] Rupprecht CE, Gibbons RV. Prophylaxis against rabies. N Engl J Med 2004;351(25): 2626–35.

[82] Coleman PG, Fevre EM, Cleaveland S. Estimating the public health impact of rabies. Emerg Infect Dis 2004;10(1):140–2.

[83] Krebs JW, Long-Marin SC, Childs JE. Causes, costs and estimates of rabies postexposure prophylaxis treatments in the United States. J Public Health Manag Pract 1998; 4(5):56–62.

[84] Warrell MJ, Warrell DA. Rabies and other lyssavirus diseases. Lancet 2004;363(9413): 959–69.

[85] Rupprecht CE, Smith JS, Krebs J, et al. Current issues in rabies prevention in the United States: health dilemmas, public coffers, private interests. Public Health Rep 1996;111(5): 400–7.

[86] Centers for Disease Control and Prevention. Rabies postexposure prophylaxis—Connecticut, 1990–1994. MMWR Morb Mortal Wkly Rep 1996;45(11):232–4.

[87] Moran GJ, Talan DA, Mower W, et al. Appropriateness of rabies postexposure prophylaxis treatment for animal exposures. JAMA 2000;284(8):1001–7.

[88] Centers for Disease Control and Prevention. Rabies prevention—United States, 1999: recommendations of the Immunization Practices Advisory Committee (ACIP). MMWR Recomm Rep 1999;48(RR–1):1–21.

[89] Noah DL, Drenzek CL, Smith JS, et al. Epidemiology of human rabies in the United States, 1980–1996. Ann Intern Med 1998;128(11):922–30.

[90] Harrigan RA, Kauffman FH. Postexposure rabies prophylaxis in an urban emergency department. J Emerg Med 1996;14(3):287–92.

[91] Vandelaer J, Birmingham M, Gasse F, et al. Tetanus in developing countries: an update on the maternal and neonatal tetanus elimination initiative. Vaccine 2003;21(24):3442–5.

[92] Edsall G. Specific prophylaxis of tetanus. JAMA 1959;171:417–27.

[93] Wassilak SGF, Roper MH, Murphy TV, et al. Tetanus toxoid. In: Plotkin SA, Orenstein WA, editors. Vaccines. Philadelphia: WB Saunders; 2004. p. 745–81.

[94] Talan DA, Abrahamian FM, Moran GJ, et al. Tetanus immunity and physician compliance with tetanus prophylaxis practices among emergency department patients presenting with wounds. Ann Emerg Med 2004;43(3):305–14.

[95] Centers for Disease Control and Prevention. Tetanus surveillance—United States, 1998–2000. MMWR Surveill Summ 2003;52(3):1–8.

[96] Centers for Disease Control and Prevention. Preventing tetanus, diphtheria, and pertussis among adults: use of tetanus toxoid, reduced diphtheria toxoid and acellular pertussis vaccine. MMWR Recomm Rep 2006;55(RR–17):1–37.

[97] Gergen PJ, McQuillan GM, Kiely M, et al. Population-based serologic survey of immunity to tetanus in the United States. N Engl J Med 1995;332(12):761–6.

[98] McQuillan GM, Kruszon-Moran D, Deforest A, et al. Serologic immunity to diphtheria and tetanus in the United States. Ann Intern Med 2002;136(9):660–6.

[99] Greco D, Salmaso S, Mastrantonio P, et al. A controlled trial of two acellular vaccines and one whole-cell vaccine against pertussis. New Engl J Med 1996;334(6):341–8.

[100] Levine L, McComb JA, Dwyer RC, et al. Active-passive tetanus immunization: choice of toxoid, dose of tetanus immune globulin and timing of injections. N Engl J Med 1966; 274(4):186–90.

[101] Strom BL, Abrutyn E, Berlin JA, et al. Dental and cardiac risk factors for infective endocarditis: a population-based, case-control study. Ann Intern Med 1998;129(10):761–9.

[102] Durack DT. Prevention of infective endocarditis. N Engl J Med 1995;332(1):38–44.

[103] Lockhart PB, Brennan MT, Fox PC, et al. Decision-making on the use of antimicrobial prophylaxis for dental procedures: a survey of infectious disease consultants and review. Clin Infect Dis 2002;34(12):1621–6.

[104] Talan DA. Prophylaxis for infective endocarditis [letter]. Ann Intern Med 1986;105(2): 299.

[105] Fitch MT, Manthey DE, McGinnis HD, et al. Abscess incision and drainage. New Engl J Med 2007;357(19):e20.

[106] Fine BC, Sheckman PR, Bartlett JC. Incision and drainage of soft tissue abscesses and bacteremia. Ann Intern Med 1985;103(4):645.

[107] Bobrow BJ, Pollack CV, Gamble S, et al. Incision and drainage of cutaneous abscesses is not associated with bacteremia in afebrile adults. Ann Emerg Med 1997;29(3):404–8.

[108] American Dental Association, American Academy of Orthopedic Surgeons. Antibiotic prophylaxis for dental patients with total joint replacements. J Am Dent Assoc 2003; 134(7):895–9.

[109] Hirota WK, Peterson K, Baron TH, et al. Guidelines for antibiotic prophylaxis for GI endoscopy. Gastrointest Endosc 2003;58(4):475–82.

[110] The Medical Letter. Antibacterial prophylaxis for dental, GI, and GU procedures. Med Lett Drugs Ther 2005;47(1213):59–60.

[111] American Urological Association, American Academy of Orthopedic Surgeons. Antibiotic prophylaxis for urological patients with total joint replacements. J Urol 2003;169(5): 1796–7.

[112] Etoch SW, Bar-Natan MF, Miller FB, et al. Tube thoracostomy: factors related to complications. Arch Surg 1995;130(5):521–5.

[113] Fallon WF Jr, Wears RL. Prophylactic antibiotics for the prevention of infectious complications including empyema following tube thoracostomy for trauma: results of meta-analysis. J Trauma 1992;33(1):110–6.

[114] Evans JT, Green JD, Carlin PE, et al. Meta-analysis of antibiotics in tube thoracostomy. Am Surg 1995;61(3):215–9.

[115] Maxwell RA, Campbell DJ, Fabian TC, et al. Use of presumptive antibiotics following tube thoracostomy for traumatic hemopneumothorax in the prevention of empyema and pneumonia: a multi-center trial. J Trauma 2004;57(4):742–8.

[116] Luchette FA, Barrie PS, Oswanski MF, et al. Practice management guidelines for prophylactic antibiotic use in tube thoracostomy for traumatic hemopneumothorax: The EAST Practice Management Guidelines Work Group. J Trauma 2000;48(4):753–7.

ELSEVIER
SAUNDERS

Infect Dis Clin N Am 22 (2008) 145–187

INFECTIOUS
DISEASE CLINICS
OF NORTH AMERICA

Biological Terrorism

Gregory J. Moran, MD, FACEP, FAAEM[a,b,c,*],
David A. Talan, MD, FACEP, FAAEM, FIDSA[a,b,c],
Fredrick M. Abrahamian, DO, FACEP[a,b]

[a]David Geffen School of Medicine at University of California Los Angeles,
Los Angeles, CA, USA
[b]Department of Emergency Medicine, Olive View-University of California Los Angeles
Medical Center, Sylmar, CA, USA
[c]Department of Medicine, Division of Infectious Diseases,
Olive View-University of California Los Angeles Medical Center, Sylmar, CA, USA

The realities of the current world situation dictate that people prepare for bioterrorism. If an attack were to occur, many people could become ill in a very short time, putting an enormous, if not overwhelming, strain on local health care facilities [1]. The emergency department will be among the first areas affected by a large influx of patients, including the truly sick and the worried well [2]. The expertise of emergency physicians and infectious disease specialists will be critical to effective planning and execution of an effective response to a bioterrorism event. Many principles used to prepare for an outbreak caused by terrorists would also be applicable to developing a response to a natural outbreak, such as an influenza pandemic (eg, Avian influenza) or severe acute respiratory syndrome epidemic [3].

Critical actions in the early stages of an event include identifying the causative agent and, if necessary, initiating infection control measures to decontaminate victims and prevent further spread of the disease [4]. Priority must be given to protecting health care workers so they can continue to care for those affected by the attack. Resources must be mobilized to increase surge capacity of emergency departments, hospitals, and clinics [5]. Large-scale vaccination programs may need to be initiated or prophylactic antibiotics distributed to a large number of individuals within a very short period.

* Corresponding author. Department of Emergency Medicine, Olive View-University of California Los Angeles Medical Center, 14445 Olive View Drive, North Annex, Sylmar, CA 91342.
E-mail address: gmoran@ucla.edu (G.J. Moran).

0891-5520/08/$ - see front matter © 2008 Elsevier Inc. All rights reserved.
doi:10.1016/j.idc.2007.12.003
id.theclinics.com

Although many potential problems associated with a bioterrorist attack seem intimidating, certain preparations could improve the ability to deal with this event. Physicians should be familiar with their contacts in the local public health department so that any suspicious illness can be reported promptly. Specific plans for bioterrorism should be incorporated in disaster planning [6]. Important topics would include infection control measures, communication with key agencies such as public health and law enforcement, mobilization of laboratory and pharmacy resources, plans for processing large numbers of patients, and increased security.

A wide range of microorganisms could potentially be used as weapons of mass destruction. The ideal agent for bioterrorism would be capable of producing illness in a large percentage of those exposed, be disseminated easily to expose large numbers of people (eg, through aerosol), remain stable and infectious despite environmental exposure, and be available to terrorists for production in adequate amounts. Fortunately, very few agents have these characteristics.

As part of their preparations for a possible bioterrorism event, the Centers for Disease Control and Prevention (CDC) have identified several organisms that are believed to have the greatest potential for use in this capacity [7]. Those believed to be top priority for preparations because of their suitability for weaponization and lethality are classified as category A agents. Several other organisms (categories B and C) are believed to be lower priority for specific preparations, but are recognized as possible bioterrorism agents. Box 1 lists the agents classified by the CDC as having potential for use in bioterrorism.

The potential for these agents to be turned into weapons varies considerably. Some are highly lethal but designated as lower-priority agents because they are unstable in the environment or would be difficult to disseminate effectively. Many of these agents cause nonlethal illness. Although highly lethal infections would create the most terror in the population, agents causing nonlethal illness could certainly provide significant social disruption, which would satisfy terrorist goals.

This article addresses some general issues related to preparing an effective response to bioterrorism. It also reviews the characteristics of organisms and toxins that could be used for bioterrorism, including clinical features, management, diagnostic testing, and infection control (Table 1).

Why biological terrorism?

Biological agents have several features that might make them more attractive to terrorists compared with conventional explosives, chemical weapons, or nuclear weapons. One advantage of biological agents is that they can inflict devastating damage even when used in minuscule amounts. They are odorless and easily concealed and are therefore difficult to detect. Enough botulinum toxin could be carried in one's pocket to kill millions of

Box 1. Agents with potential for use in biological terrorism

Category A

Easy to disseminate; cause high morbidity and mortality; and
require specific enhancements of CDC's diagnostic capacity
and enhanced disease surveillance
   Anthrax
   Plague
   Smallpox
   Hemorrhagic Fevers
   Botulism
   Tularemia

Category B

Somewhat easy to disseminate; cause moderate morbidity and
low mortality; and require specific enhancements of CDC's
diagnostic capacity and enhanced disease surveillance
   Coxiella burnetii (Q fever)
   Brucella species (brucellosis)
   Burkholderia mallei (glanders)
   Alphaviruses
   Venezuelan encephalomyelitis
   Eastern and Western equine encephalomyelitis
   Ricin toxin from *Ricinus communis* (castor beans)
   Epsilon toxin of *Clostridium perfringens*
   Staphylococcus enterotoxin B
   Food or waterborne agents
   Salmonella species
   Shigella dysenteriae
   Escherichia coli O157:H7
   Vibrio cholerae
   Cryptosporidium parvum

Category C

Emerging pathogens that could be engineered for mass
dissemination in the future because of availability; ease of
production and dissemination; and potential for high morbidity
and mortality and major health impact
   Nipah virus
   Hantaviruses
   Tickborne hemorrhagic fever viruses
   Tickborne encephalitis viruses
   Yellow fever
   Multidrug-resistant tuberculosis

Table 1
Agents of bioterrorism

Disease	Clinical presentation	Diagnostic tests	Person-to-person transmission	Treatment	Vaccine/prophylaxis
Anthrax	Inhalation: fever, malaise for 1–2 days followed by respiratory distress, shock May have meningitis. Highly fatal if untreated Cutaneous: red papule progressing to shallow ulcer or blister, then black eschar	CXR may show wide mediastinum Gram-positive bacilli in blood, CSF, or skin lesion CSF may be bloody Blood culture is highest yield for inhalation anthrax	No	Ciprofloxacin or Doxycycline plus one to two other drugs Other active drugs include penicillin, clindamycin, rifampin, vancomycin, imipenem Levofloxacin or moxifloxacin probably also effective	Prophylaxis: ciprofloxacin or doxycycline for 60 days (30 days if given with vaccine) Bioport vaccine 0.5 mL SC at 0, 2, 4 weeks, 6, 12, 18 months, then annual boosters
Botulism	Cranial nerve palsies (particularly involving eyes) progressing to descending paralysis Paralysis lasts for weeks to months.	Diagnosis mostly clinical Mouse bioassay using patient serum takes several days, not widely available	No	Primarily ventilator support Antitoxin can prevent further progression, but will not reverse paralysis	None
Brucellosis	Fever, chills, anorexia, malaise May last weeks to months	Blood culture (slow-growing; notify laboratory if suspected) or serology Leukocyte counts variable CXR nonspecific	No Culture specimens may pose risk to laboratory workers	doxycycline or fluoroquinolone plus rifampin	doxycycline or fluoroquinolone plus rifampin for 6 weeks No vaccine available

Disease	Symptoms	Diagnosis	Contagious / Isolation	Treatment	Prophylaxis
Cholera	Severe watery diarrhea	Stool culture with special media	Rare Use body fluid precautions	Fluids, ciprofloxacin or doxycycline	Prophylaxis: ciprofloxacin or doxycycline Two-dose vaccine, not highly effective
Glanders (*Burkholderia mallei*)	Tender skin nodules, septicemia, pneumonia	Serology (not widely available) Blood culture often negative	Low risk, but respiratory isolation recommended Culture specimens may pose risk to laboratory workers	Doxycycline, TMP/SMX, chloramphenicol, fluoroquinolones, or aminoglycosides	Doxycycline, TMP/SMX, macrolides, or fluoroquinolones can be used for prophylaxis No vaccine
Pneumonic plague	Fever, chills, malaise, cough, respiratory distress, hemoptysis, meningitis, sepsis Highly fatal if untreated	Gram-negative coccobacilli in blood, sputum, lymph node aspirate Safety-pin appearance with Wright or Giemsa stain ELISA antigen test and serology using ELISA or IFA also available	High risk Use respiratory droplet isolation	Streptomycin, gentamicin, doxycycline, or chloramphenicol	Doxycycline or quinolone for 6 days Killed vaccine for bubonic plague, not effective against aerosol exposure (no longer manufactured)
Q fever (*Coxiella burnetii*)	Fever, chills, headache, sometimes pneumonia Mortality is low	Serology Titers may not be elevated until 2–3 weeks into illness	No Culture or tissue specimens may pose risk to lab workers.	Tetracycline or doxycycline	Tetracycline or doxycycline for 5 days for prophylaxis. Single dose inactivated whole cell vaccine, not licensed in United States
Ricin	Fever, dyspnea, vomiting, diarrhea, shock	CXR may show pulmonary edema Serology (not widely available)	No	Supportive	No vaccine or prophylaxis available

(continued on next page)

Table 1 (continued)

Disease	Clinical presentation	Diagnostic tests	Person-to-person transmission	Treatment	Vaccine/prophylaxis
Smallpox	Fever, malaise, headache for 1–2 days, followed by papular rash progressing to vesicles and pustules.	Scabs or pustular fluid can be forwarded to CDC through local public health dept. Can test vesicular fluid locally to exclude varicella	High risk Use strict respiratory isolation Identify any possible contacts Specimens can pose risk to laboratory workers	Supportive Cidofovir may be useful, but not tested	Vaccinia vaccine can prevent illness in contacts up to several days after exposure
Staphylococcal enterotoxin B	Sudden onset of fever, headache, myalgias, vomiting, diarrhea, dry cough Usually resolves within a day	Urine antigen, ELISA of nasal swab (not widely available)	No	Supportive	No vaccine
Tularemia	Fever, malaise, prostration, headache, weight loss and non-productive cough	CXR may show infiltrate, hilar adenopathy, or effusion Culture and gram stain of blood or sputum may show small, faintly staining, slow growing gram-negative coccobacilli. Serology usually positive after 1–2 weeks	No Culture specimens may pose risk to laboratory workers	Streptomycin, gentamicin, doxycycline, chloramphenicol, or fluoroquinolones	Doxycycline or ciprofloxacin for 14 days Investigational live attenuated vaccine

Disease	Clinical features	Diagnosis	Transmission/Isolation	Treatment	Prophylaxis/Vaccine
Venezuelan, Eastern, or Western equine encephalitis	Most have mild syndrome of fever, headache, and myalgia. Rarely progresses to encephalitis	Serology of CSF or serum	Only via vector. Isolation not necessary	Supportive	Inactive vaccines for VEE, EEE, WEE are poorly effective. Live vaccine for VEE has high incidence of side effects
Viral hemorrhagic fevers (eg. Ebola)	Fever, prostration, myalgia, conjunctival injection, petechial rash, bleeding. Most are highly fatal	Thrombocytopenia. Identification of virus requires special testing at CDC	Moderate risk. Primarily transmitted through body fluids, but strict respiratory isolation is recommended	Primarily supportive. Ribavirin may be effective for some, including Congo-Crimean HF, Lassa fever	No prophylaxis or vaccine available

Abbreviations: CDC, Centers for Disease Control and Prevention; CSF, cerebrospinal fluid; CXR, chest x-ray; EEE, Eastern equine encephalomyelitis; ELISA, enzyme-linked immunosorbent assay; HF, hemorrhagic fever; IFA, indirect fluorescent antibody; SC, subcutaneous; TMP/SMX, trimethoprim-sulfamethoxazole; VEE, Venezuelan equine encephalomyelitis; WEE, Western equine encephalomyelitis.

people if properly dispersed. Because biological agents do not trigger metal detectors, a terrorist could board a commercial airplane and transport the agent to any city in the world, where civilian populations are largely unprotected from this kind of attack.

Although access to hazardous biological agents is now more restricted than in the past, many agents are easy to obtain, certainly much more so than materials such as plutonium that could be used for other weapons of mass destruction. A biological weapon may be more difficult to prepare than a simple pipe bomb, but could often be prepared with only basic microbiology skills. Biological agents are also more difficult to trace because there is a delay between release of the agent and the first development of symptoms. A terrorist could release a biological agent in a major metropolitan area and be on another continent before anyone knows an attack occurred.

Biological agents certainly have the capacity to produce terror. Even if only a few people actually become ill, an entire city (or even country) could be disrupted if people believe they have been exposed to a deadly organism, such as Ebola virus or plague. In addition to preparing for the medical emergency, preparing for the panic and chaos that a bioterrorism attack would cause is also important. Thousands of people, ill or healthy, could descend on emergency departments and clinics, convinced they are about to die.

Probable scenarios and likely problems

One possible scenario for a large-scale biological attack would be aerosolized dispersal of a biological agent, such as from an airplane flying over a populated area or a small device planted in a ventilation system or crowded location. Fortunately, very few biological agents remain infectious after prolonged exposure to air and sunlight, making a large-scale attack difficult.

Because most illnesses caused by biological agents involve incubation periods, several days are likely to elapse before people become sick. In addition, because the victims will probably seek medical care at different facilities, some time may pass before the medical community is even aware that anything unusual has occurred. The epidemiologic pattern could be an early sign that an attack has occurred, but with patients presenting at different locations, often with relatively nonspecific signs and symptoms, suspecting that an act of terrorism has occurred will be difficult until the number of victims becomes significant.

In addition to the challenge of treating illnesses, clinicians will be faced with serious logistical problems if they receive a multitude of victims. Personnel, medications, and other resources are likely to be insufficient [8]. Prophylactic therapies are effective against some biological agents. However, knowing that doxycycline or ciprofloxacin can prevent illness in people exposed to anthrax will not help when immediate demand exceeds available supply. The federal government has stockpiles of antibiotics, as do many large cities, but rapid distribution to large numbers of people will be difficult. Shortages of medicine could exacerbate the panic and chaos caused by the attack, not only among the victims streaming into emergency departments and hospitals but also among health care personnel.

Because some of the diseases caused by biological agents can be spread person-to-person, isolation of victims may be necessary, which will be another formidable challenge, especially with thousands of victims [9]. Many facilities do not have enough isolation beds even for their current needs [10], so patients will probably have to be cohorted in designated wards. Use of portable high-efficiency particulate air (HEPA) filters may also be useful in an outbreak situation [11].

Emergency department surveillance for bioterrorism events

As the front line of clinical medicine, emergency departments are key to an effective surveillance program [12]. Emergency physicians (and infectious disease specialists) must continue to be on the lookout for unusual syndromes or clusters of illness that could represent a natural or intentional outbreak.

Surveillance systems have been greatly expanded in recent years in response to concerns about bioterrorism. Many emergency departments are now part of regional syndromic surveillance systems [13]. Computerized emergency department information systems that continuously collect information have facilitated inclusion of many facilities in these types of systems and facilitate surveillance with minimal resource commitment. Systems that require human involvement to actively collect data or enter it into a dedicated system are likely to be abandoned or become less effective after many years of data collection with no real events [14]. Systems that run continuously in the background are more efficient and allow generation of data on the background incidence and variability of different clinical syndromes. Additional benefits of these systems include improved recognition of naturally occurring outbreaks and facilitation of research with large emergency department databases. These systems are generally designed so that individual patient identifiers are not sent to the central database, but public health reporting is exempted from Health Insurance Portability and Accountability Act (HIPAA) requirements for patient consent to share information [15].

Although syndromic surveillance systems could be useful in detecting disease outbreaks, the usefulness of these systems is unproven. Syndromic surveillance has been found to correlate with activity of some common viruses, such as influenza and respiratory syncytial virus (RSV) [16], but the more difficult task of detecting the first cases of a new outbreak has not been seen. Even with these surveillance systems in place, the initial detection of a bioterrorism event may still result from laboratory identification of anthrax, smallpox, plague, or Ebola virus. It is unlikely that any syndromic surveillance system would have detected the United States mail-related anthrax cases of 2001 before the first case was identified through laboratory testing of cerebrospinal fluid (CSF). Unfortunately, microbiologic identification in the laboratory usually takes a couple of days, during which the outbreak may spread beyond easy containment. Investing in rapid laboratory testing methods that could be performed during emergency department evaluation might improve early detection. The real test will be when the next outbreak or bioterrorism event occurs.

The presence of syndromic surveillance systems does not remove the obligation of individual physicians to be vigilant for unusual clinical presentations and notify the local public health department if an infectious disease is suspected that could pose a threat to public health.

Agents with potential use as biological weapons

Some biological agents can be fatal, such as anthrax, botulinum toxin, and the viruses that cause hemorrhagic fevers, but terrorists could also meet their goals simply through making many people ill. Diseases such as brucellosis and tularemia are rarely lethal but can wreak havoc in a community if enough people are afflicted.

Fortunately, most biological agents cannot be dispersed effectively through aerosol. Many are not stable enough to withstand temperature changes, exposure to sunlight, and drying. Anthrax is often cited as an agent likely to be used for bioterrorism because spores are stable for many years, even in extreme environments. The spores are also of an optimal size (1–2 μm), which allows them to be inhaled into the lungs and deposited in the alveolar spaces. Most viral agents, such as those that cause hemorrhagic fevers and encephalitis, are unstable and therefore would be difficult to disperse through aerosolized large-scale attacks, but smallpox virus can remain viable after many years of storage. Bacterial agents vary in their stability during storage and dispersal. Although toxins such as botulinum toxin and staphylococcal enterotoxin B can remain stable for many years in storage, they can be difficult to disperse effectively to cause illness in a large population.

The agents designated by the CDC as category A are believed to be the greatest threat because of ease of dissemination or transmission, high mortality rate, potential major impact on public health, ability to incite panic and social disruption, and the requirement for additional major public health preparedness measures (see Box 1).

Category B agents would be moderately easy to disseminate, would cause moderate morbidity and low mortality, and would require specific enhancements of the CDC's diagnostic capacity and disease surveillance capabilities. The agents classified by the CDC as category C are emerging pathogens that could someday be engineered for mass exposure because of availability, ease of production and dissemination, and potential for high morbidity and mortality. Preparedness for category C agents requires ongoing research to improve disease detection, diagnosis, treatment, and prevention. Which newly emergent pathogens terrorists might use is impossible to know in advance.

For detection and response to these agents, a strong public health infrastructure is essential. It is also important for physicians to notify the local health department if unusual patterns of illness are observed.

Category A agents

Anthrax

History and significance

Bacillus anthracis could be considered to be the perfect agent for bioterrorism. It occurs naturally as a zoonotic disease of persons who handle contaminated animal products, such as hair or hides. It forms spores that are stable over long periods and can withstand exposure to air, sunlight, and even some disinfectants. Anthrax was studied as a possible weapon by the United States when it had an active biological weapons program, and has been weaponized by other countries [17]. Anthrax bacteria are easy to cultivate in the microbiology laboratory and can be readily induced to produce spores. The Soviet Union produced weaponized anthrax in ton quantities during the cold war era. An outbreak of inhalational anthrax occurred near a Soviet bioweapons facility at Sverdlovsk in 1979, resulting in 77 infections and 66 deaths, with some victims becoming ill up to 6 weeks after exposure [18]. The Japanese cult group Aum Shinrikyo attempted several attacks with anthrax in the 1990s but were unsuccessful [19].

Anthrax became the most notorious bioterrorism agent after October 4, 2001, when a 63-year-old man died of inhalational anthrax that was traced to intentional exposure through the United States mail [20,21]. This instance represented the first inhalation anthrax case in the United States since 1976 [22]. Ultimately, 18 cases of anthrax (11 inhalational and 7 cutaneous) were confirmed. More than 30,000 people who were potentially exposed received postexposure prophylaxis, and none developed inhalational anthrax.

Clinical presentation

Anthrax can present as three distinct clinical syndromes in humans: cutaneous, inhalation, and gastrointestinal. Cutaneous anthrax, the most common naturally occurring form, is usually spread through contact with infected animals, particularly cows, sheep, and horses, or their products. Cutaneous anthrax (Fig. 1) typically produces large black eschars on the skin, but in early stages may appear as papules that progress to vesicles. Patients may also experience lymphadenopathy, fever, malaise, and nausea. Local cutaneous anthrax has a mortality rate of less than 1% if treated but can occasionally become systemic, with mortality rates approaching 20% [23].

Gastrointestinal anthrax is rare in humans. It is acquired by ingesting inadequately cooked meat from infected animals. As the ingested spores germinate, the infected person may develop ulcers in the mouth or esophagus, or may develop lesions lower in the intestinal tract that caused them to

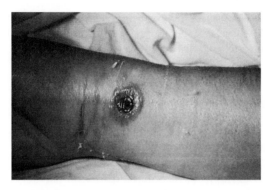

Fig. 1. Anthrax skin lesion. (*Courtesy of* Centers for Disease Control and Prevention/Dr. Philip S. Brachman.)

present with abdominal pain, fever, and diarrhea that progresses to a sepsis syndrome with high mortality.

A far greater threat is posed by the inhalational form of anthrax. This type of anthrax, also known as woolsorter's disease when it occurs naturally, is only rarely seen among wool or tannery workers, but is the form of anthrax most likely to be spread through a terrorist attack. Inhalational anthrax can be rapidly fatal once symptoms begin.

The victims of the 2001 anthrax attack presented with a fairly consistent clinical syndrome [24–26]. Symptoms began as a nonspecific prodrome resembling influenza, with malaise, dry cough, and mild fever. This progressed to chills, sweats, nausea, and vomiting, with development of chest pain and respiratory distress. Almost all patients had some abnormality on chest radiograph or CT scans, including infiltrates, pleural effusion, or mediastinal widening. Some patients developed meningitis. Inhalation anthrax can sometimes present without the usual symptoms of chest pain and shortness of breath [27]. The illness often progressed to septic shock and death approximately 24 to 36 hours after the appearance of respiratory distress.

Before the events of 2001 in the United States, almost all cases of inhalational anthrax were fatal when treatment was initiated after development of significant symptoms. The case fatality rate was 45% among the 11 confirmed inhalational cases resulting from bioterrorism in the fall of 2001, largely attributed to earlier and more aggressive supportive care and antibiotic therapy [22,28].

Diagnosis

Generally, diagnosis must be suspected on clinical grounds for treatment to be initiated in time to be beneficial. By the time the disease is confirmed through laboratory tests, many patients will be beyond help [29]. *B anthracis* is detectable through Gram stain of the blood and blood culture on routine media, but often not until the patient is seriously ill. An enzyme-linked immunosorbent assay (ELISA) for the anthrax toxin exists, but most hospital laboratories do not have it readily available. The organism may also be identified in CSF, because approximately 50% of cases have hemorrhagic meningitis [30]. Chest films may show a widened mediastinum and pleural effusions [31], but those findings are not universal and are usually seen late in the disease.

Infection control precautions

Anthrax does not spread person-to-person, and standard precautions are recommended. However, persons who present shortly after exposure may still be contaminated with spores. Any persons coming into direct contact with a substance alleged to be anthrax spores should simply bathe with soap and water and store contaminated clothing in a plastic bag, but decontamination procedures for other persons in the area should not be necessary. Disinfectants such as bleach solutions can be used to decontaminate inanimate objects, but are not recommended for skin.

Treatment and prophylaxis

The mainstay of treatment is antibiotic therapy, but the regimen should be started as early as possible to be effective. Although penicillin is usually regarded as the preferred treatment for naturally occurring anthrax [32], penicillin-resistant strains are known to occur, and the belief is that terrorists would be likely to use a more resistant strain (although this was not the case in the 2001 attack). Penicillin is not recommended as empiric treatment until susceptibility of the organism is known. *B anthracis* is also susceptible to tetracyclines, erythromycin, chloramphenicol, gentamicin, and fluoroquinolones. Initial empiric treatment with ciprofloxacin or another fluoroquinolone is recommended until susceptibility is known [33]. Supportive therapy to maintain the airway, replenish fluids, and alleviate shock is also crucial. Because spores can be dormant for a long time, a 60-day course of antibiotics is recommended for treating anthrax.

In patients who were exposed to anthrax but are not yet sick, illness and death can be prevented with prophylactic antibiotics. The CDC recommends ciprofloxacin (500 mg orally twice daily) or doxycycline (100 mg orally twice daily) as first-line prophylaxis after inhalational exposure to anthrax, and for presumptive treatment of mild symptoms after anthrax exposure. If anthrax exposure is confirmed, antibiotics should be continued for at least 60 days in all exposed individuals, and patients should be followed up closely after antibiotics are discontinued.

A vaccine for anthrax, derived from an attenuated anthrax strain, has been licensed by the U.S. Food and Drug Administration since 1970 [34]. This vaccine has been used mostly for military personnel, and might not be generally available to the public in adequate amounts in the event of a large biological attack. The vaccine is given repeatedly in a series of six subcutaneous injections over 18 months and can cause several adverse effects [35]. It is not licensed for use against inhalational anthrax exposure, but some limited animal data suggest protection [36]. Attempts to develop a better vaccine have met with technical problems and political interference [37].

Several anthrax hoaxes have been perpetrated in many United States cities, both before and after the 2001 attacks. Public health officials, working with law enforcement and first-response personnel, should determine the necessity for decontamination and prophylactic therapy after these alleged exposures. Until the substance can be identified, chemoprophylaxis is a reasonable precaution if the threat is credible. Good communication among public health, law enforcement, and clinicians caring for persons who may have been exposed is critical for appropriate management.

Plague

History and significance

Few illnesses carry as many terrifying connotations for the general public as plague, caused by the gram-negative bacillus *Yersinia pestis*. The "Black Death" killed millions of people throughout Europe in the fourteenth century. A more recent pandemic originated in China and spread worldwide at the turn of the twentieth century. Bubonic plague is the most common naturally occurring form. It is a zoonotic infection spread from the rodent reservoir to man through the bites of infected fleas. Plague, like anthrax, also has a pneumonic form, which can be transmitted through inhalation of droplets spread by cough or, in the event of a terrorist attack, through inhalation of an aerosol containing *Y pestis*. As with anthrax, the pneumonic form of the disease is far more dangerous. Left untreated, pneumonic plague is nearly always fatal within 2 days of onset of symptoms.

Plague is more difficult to use as a biological weapon than anthrax because *Y pestis* is susceptible to drying, heat, and ultraviolet light. However, unlike anthrax, secondary cases may result from person-to-person transmission. Attempts to use plague as a biological weapon date back to the ancient practice of flinging plague-infected corpses over the walls of cities under siege. The Japanese attempted to use plague as a biological weapon by releasing infected fleas over cities in Manchuria during World War II, but dissemination attempts met with limited success. The United States did not develop plague as a potential weapon because of its persistence in the environment and the possibility of noncombatant and friendly casualties after an attack. The Soviet Union reportedly developed dry, antibiotic-resistant, environmentally stable forms of *Y pestis* that could be disseminated as an aerosol [38].

Clinical presentation

Bubonic plague begins as painful adenopathy several days after the infecting flea bite. Without treatment, the illness progresses within several days to septicemia. Approximately 5% to 15% of patients will develop a secondary pneumonia that can spread plague through droplets from coughing.

Aerosol dispersal with resulting pneumonic plague would be more likely in a bioterrorism attack. After an incubation period of 2 to 3 days, patients who have pneumonic plague typically develop fulminant pneumonia, with malaise, high fever, cough, hemoptysis, and septicemia with ecchymoses and extremity necrosis. Findings on chest radiographs are generally typical of patients who have pneumonia. The disease progresses rapidly, leading to dyspnea, stridor, cyanosis, and septic shock. Death is normally the result of respiratory failure and circulatory collapse [39].

Diagnosis

A presumptive diagnosis can often be made by identifying *Y pestis* in Gram's, Wayson's, or Wright-Giemsa stain of blood, sputum, or lymph node aspirate samples. A definitive diagnosis is generally made with culture studies. An ELISA test for plague exists, but it is not widely available. Direct fluorescent antibody staining of the capsular antigen is also available. Buboes may be aspirated with a small-gauge needle, but incision and drainage should not be performed because of the risk for aerosolization of the organism. The organism has a characteristic bipolar "safety pin" appearance.

Hematologic studies will show leukocytosis with left shift. Bilirubin levels and serum aminotransferases are often elevated. Antibody studies are not useful for diagnosing disease during the acute phase. Blood, sputum, bubo aspirate, and CSF cultures on normal blood agar media are often negative at 24 hours but positive by 48 hours. The colonies of *Y pestis* are usually 1 to 3 mm in diameter and have been described as having a "beaten copper" or "hammered metal" appearance [36].

Infection control precautions

Unlike pulmonary anthrax, pneumonic plague is very contagious. Strict respiratory isolation is necessary until infected patients have undergone treatment for at least 3 days. Unfortunately, because the initial presentation resembles that of severe pneumonia caused by other agents, the actual diagnosis may not be known for several days. Therefore, patients who present with fulminant pneumonia after a suspected biological attack should be held in respiratory isolation until the cause has been determined.

Treatment and prophylaxis

Early treatment with antibiotics, within 24 hours of the appearance of symptoms, is crucial to the survival of patients who have pneumonic plague. Streptomycin is the traditional preferred agent but may not be readily available in some facilities. Doxycycline, gentamicin, ceftriaxone, chloramphenicol, and fluoroquinolones should also be effective. Treatment should be continued for a minimum of 10 days, or for 4 days after clinical recovery. Patients who have mild illness can be treated with oral doxycycline or fluoroquinolones.

Persons exposed to plague should receive postexposure prophylaxis with doxycycline (100 mg twice daily) or a fluoroquinolone for 6 days. Medical personnel who practice good infection control precautions should not require prophylaxis. A recombinant vaccine is under development and seems to protect against pneumonic plague.

Smallpox

History and significance

Smallpox (variola) is a DNA orthopoxvirus that has been a scourge to humans throughout recorded history. No nonhuman reservoirs or human carriers exist for smallpox; the disease survives through continual person-to-person transmission. The first documented epidemic of smallpox was during the Egyptian-Hittite war in 1350 BC. The mummy of Ramses V has lesions that suggest he died of smallpox at the age of 35 years in 1143 BC. Smallpox was used inadvertently as a biological weapon when Cortez introduced it to the new world in 1520, devastating much of the native population. The English used smallpox intentionally during the French and Indian war in 1754 when tainted blankets were distributed to Native Americans, with up to 50% mortality in many tribes. The last case of wild smallpox occurred in Somalia in 1977, although a few small outbreaks have occurred related to laboratory exposure. The disease was declared eradicated by the World Health Organization (WHO) in 1980 and routine vaccination was stopped soon after.

Because of its propensity for secondary human-to-human transmission, smallpox is one of the most feared agents that could be unleashed in a biological attack [40]. Because vaccination is no longer given, most persons today are susceptible to infection. Even those who were vaccinated as children are likely to be susceptible, because immunity wanes over time.

Stocks of variola virus are supposedly stored at only two WHO-approved storage facilities: the CDC in Atlanta and the NPO (Scientific and Production Association) in the Novosibirsk region of Russia. The Soviet Union may have developed stockpiles of weaponized smallpox and experimented with genetic manipulation of the virus [38]. Many believe that some virus samples may be in the hands of potential terrorists. Because the virus is difficult to obtain, an intentional smallpox exposure would require extensive resources that might be out of reach for small groups.

Clinical presentation

The incubation period associated with smallpox is approximately 12 days. Smallpox begins with a febrile prodrome a few days before the rash that may also be accompanied by chills, head and body aches, nausea, vomiting, and abdominal pain [41]. The characteristic rash develops on the extremities and spreads centrally. Skin lesions evolve slowly from macules to papules to vesicles to pustules, with each stage lasting 1 to 2 days. Unlike chickenpox, all smallpox lesions are at the same stage of development.

The first lesions are often on the oral mucosa or palate, face, or forearms. The vesicles or pustules tend to be distributed centrifugally, with the greatest concentration on the face and distal extremities, including the palms and soles. Vesicles and pustules are deep-seated, firm, or hard, round, well-circumscribed lesions; they are sharply raised and feel like small round objects embedded under the skin (Fig. 2). As they evolve, the lesions may become umbilicated or confluent and will scab over in 1 to 2 weeks, leaving hypopigmented scars.

If a biological attack is not known to have occurred, some early smallpox cases are likely to be mistaken for chickenpox or other diseases. Chickenpox differs from smallpox in that the prodrome is milder, the vesicles are superficial (ie, easily collapse on puncture) and predominate on the trunk as opposed to the distal extremities, and active and healing lesions occur simultaneously.

Mortality is reported as approximately 30% overall among unvaccinated persons, but this reflects historical data in populations without modern medical care. Mortality is higher in infants and elderly individuals, and would likely be much lower among healthy adults and older children. Death occurs late in the first week or during the second week of the illness and is caused by the toxemia induced by the overwhelming viremia. A rare hemorrhagic form occurs with extensive bleeding into the skin and gastrointestinal tract followed almost universally by death within a few days.

Diagnosis

The diagnosis of smallpox can be confirmed with electron microscopy or gel diffusion on vesicular scrapings, but these modalities are not available in most hospital laboratories. If smallpox is suspected, the laboratory must be notified to take proper precautions. Smallpox specimens should be handled under biosafety level 4 conditions. Because testing for varicella virus is usually available, a vesicular eruption in which varicella cannot be identified should alert clinicians to possible smallpox. Specimens could then be forwarded for testing at a specialized laboratory, such as at the CDC or U.S.

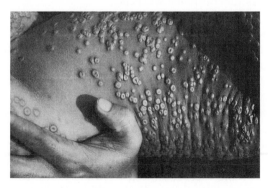

Fig. 2. Smallpox skin lesions on the trunk. (*Courtesy of* Centers for Disease Control and Prevention/James Hicks.)

Army Medical Research Institute of Infectious Diseases (USAMRIID). Electron microscopy cannot reliably differentiate between variola, vaccinia (cowpox), and monkeypox. New polymerase chain reaction (PCR) techniques that can rapidly diagnose smallpox may soon be available.

Infection control precautions

Identification of even a single case of smallpox would signal an infectious disease emergency of worldwide significance. Clinicians who suspect smallpox should immediately contact their local health department and their hospital infection control officer. The local health department will immediately contact the state public health department and the CDC. The most important issue concerning smallpox would be containment of any subsequent outbreak. If an initial outbreak cannot be contained within a single community, an arduous worldwide eradication effort may need to be begun anew.

Smallpox is readily transmitted person-to-person through respiratory droplets. Because delays in the initial diagnosis are likely, some secondary exposures may already have occurred by the time smallpox virus is identified as the cause of illness. Although people are generally not considered infectious until the rash begins, they can shed virus in early stages of the rash before it can be readily identified as smallpox.

Aggressive quarantine measures will be necessary to prevent further spread. Anyone who has had direct contact with an infected person should undergo strict quarantine with respiratory isolation for 17 days. In large-scale outbreaks, infected individuals may need to be kept at home.

Virions can also remain viable on fomites for up to 1 week. All laundry, including bedding of infected individuals, should be autoclaved or washed in hot water with bleach. Standard hospital antiviral surface cleaners are adequate for disinfecting surfaces (eg, counters, floors). Viable virus has been found in scabs that have been stored for up to 13 years, so meticulous decontamination is crucial. If possible, all bodies should be cremated to prevent subsequent exposure of individuals who have had contact with the deceased, such as funeral home workers.

Treatment and prophylaxis

No known effective treatment exists against smallpox. The drug cidofovir, used to treat cytomegalovirus infections, may be active against variola virus, but no data currently show the drug's efficacy in humans. Management of cases will be largely supportive care.

A vaccine based on the vaccinia virus is effective for immunizing against smallpox, and has been the mainstay of smallpox control. Unlike many other vaccines, smallpox vaccine can be effective in preventing disease even up to several days after exposure. Although stockpiles of the vaccine were low after routine vaccination ceased in the 1980s, concern about bioterrorism has prompted recent development of more modern vaccine manufacturing methods and creation of new stockpiles.

Smallpox vaccination is not without risk [42]. Risks are higher for those who have never been previously vaccinated. Complications from the use of the current smallpox (vaccinia) vaccine range from the relatively benign autoinoculation and generalized vaccinia through the more severe progressive vaccinia. The most serious complications include postvaccinial encephalopathy and encephalitis, but fortunately these are rare [43]. Because vaccinia is a live virus, potential exists for secondary transmission after vaccination [44]. In the era of routine smallpox eradication, the only contraindications to vaccination were pregnancy, certain immunocompromised conditions, and eczema. In the setting of a bioterrorism-related smallpox outbreak, those believed to have been exposed to the virus would have no absolute contraindications to vaccination.

In 2002, president Bush announced a program for the vaccination of health care workers against smallpox. The goal was to vaccinate 500,000 health care workers, but only a very small number actually received the vaccine. Many health care workers declined vaccination because of concerns about adverse reactions [45]. An advisory panel recommended against routine vaccination of emergency physicians because of concern that even a small risk for adverse reactions outweighed the minimal benefit that could be expected from smallpox vaccination in the absence of smallpox transmission anywhere in the world [46]. In the event of even a single smallpox case or a credible imminent threat, the benefits of smallpox vaccination would become clearer. Performing a rigorous scientific analysis of the risks and benefits for smallpox vaccination is impossible, because the true risk of a smallpox attack is unknown. The probability that any individual physician would be among those to see the first few cases of a smallpox outbreak is extremely low. Because smallpox vaccine can provide protection up to several days after exposure, a strategy to ensure timely vaccination of exposed health care workers and the general public if a smallpox case is identified would avoid the risk for unnecessary adverse reactions to smallpox vaccine while smallpox does not exist. Emergency and infectious disease physicians should work with public health authorities to ensure that these mechanisms are in place.

The Advisory Committee on Immunization Practices (ACIP) and the Health care Infection Control Practices Advisory Committee (HICPAC) recommend that each acute-care hospital identify health care workers who can be vaccinated and trained to provide direct medical care for the first smallpox patients requiring hospital admission and to evaluate and manage patients who are suspected as having smallpox [47]. When feasible, the first-stage vaccination program should include previously vaccinated health care personnel to decrease the potential for adverse events. Additionally, persons administering smallpox vaccine in this pre-event vaccination program should be vaccinated.

Smallpox vaccine is administered by using the multiple-puncture technique with a bifurcated needle packaged with the vaccine and diluent. According to the product labeling, 2 to 3 punctures are recommended for primary vaccination and 15 for revaccination. A trace of blood should appear at the vaccination site after 15 to 20 seconds; if no trace of blood is visible, an additional 3 insertions should be made by using the same bifurcated needle without reinserting the needle into the vaccine vial. If no evidence of vaccine take is apparent after 7 days, the person can be vaccinated again. Optimal infection-control practices and appropriate site care should prevent transmission of vaccinia virus from vaccinated health care workers to patients. Health care personnel providing direct patient care should keep their vaccination sites covered with gauze in combination with a semipermeable membrane dressing to absorb exudates and provide a barrier for containment of vaccinia virus to minimize the risk of transmission. The dressing should also be covered by a layer of clothing [48].

Viral hemorrhagic fevers

History and significance

Like plague, the viral hemorrhagic fevers, which include Ebola and Marburg disease, Lassa fever, and Bolivian hemorrhagic fever, incite fear in the general public. Many of these viruses cause rapidly progressive illnesses that carry extremely high mortality rates. Viral hemorrhagic fevers can be spread in various ways. Lassa fever, for instance, is usually spread through the ingestion of food contaminated with rodent urine, although person-to-person transmission through contact with urine, feces, or saliva can also occur.

Yellow fever and dengue (Flaviviridae) are probably the archetypical diseases of this group but are not considered significant bioterrorism threat agents. Hantavirus (Bunyaviridae) is enzootic in rodents. West Africa's Lassa fever, and Argentine, Bolivian, Brazilian, and Venezuelan hemorrhagic fevers (Arenaviridae) are also enzootic in rodents within their respective areas. The most publicized viral hemorrhagic fevers are the Ebola and Marburg (Filoviridae) viruses. These viruses produce grotesquely lethal diseases, making them favorites with the popular media. The reservoir and natural transmission of Ebola and Marburg are unknown, but they are readily transmittable through infected blood and tissue. Aerosols may be formed naturally when infectious body fluids are expelled or, in the case of hantavirus, when rodent feces and urine are resuspended from movement in the area. Laboratory cultures can yield sufficient concentrations of organisms to provide a credible terrorist weapon if disseminated as an aerosol [36].

Clinical presentation

The clinical presentations of different viral hemorrhagic fevers vary, but all can involve diffuse hemorrhage and bleeding diatheses. The incubation periods of the hemorrhagic fevers range from 4 to 21 days. The more severe fevers, such as Ebola, generally have shorter incubation periods. Patients typically present with a nonspecific prodrome that includes fever, myalgia, and prostration. On physical examination, the only findings may be conjunctival injection, mild hypotension, flushing, and scattered petechiae.

Laboratory testing may show thrombocytopenia or other signs of disseminated intravascular coagulation or elevated levels of liver enzymes or creatinine. Within hours or days after the initial presentation, patients will experience a quick deterioration of their status, followed by mucous membrane hemorrhage and shock, often with signs of neurologic, pulmonary, and hepatic involvement [49].

Diagnosis

Specific tests for some hemorrhagic fevers exist but are not available at most hospital laboratories. Specific identification requires ELISA detection of antiviral IgM antibodies or direct culture of the viral agent from blood or tissue samples. These tests can only be performed at specialized laboratories, such as those available at CDC or USAMRIID. If the agent remains unknown, it may be visualized through electron microscopy (Fig. 3) followed by immunohistochemical techniques. The laboratory should be notified if Ebola or Marburg viruses are suspected because specimens should be handled under biosafety level 4 precautions.

Infection control precautions

Contact precautions are necessary for all health care personnel managing persons who have hemorrhagic fever [50]. All body fluids should be considered infectious. In several outbreaks in Africa, hospital personnel were able to prevent transmission to themselves and other patients simply through wearing gowns, gloves, and masks. Respiratory isolation, however, may be necessary for patients who experience massive hemorrhage into the lungs. Aerosol transmission of hemorrhagic fever has been shown in animal studies but does not appear to be a significant mode among humans. Under ideal conditions, each patient should be cared for in a private room. The room should be entered through an adjoining anteroom that is used for decontamination and hand washing.

Treatment and prophylaxis

Good supportive care is the mainstay of therapy for patients who have any viral hemorrhagic fever. Special care must be taken during fluid

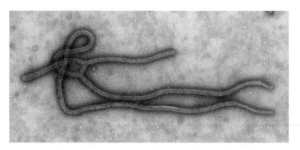

Fig. 3. Electron micrograph of Ebola virus. (*Courtesy of* Centers for Disease Control and Prevention/Cynthia Goldsmith.)

resuscitation, because fluid transudation into the lungs will occur in some patients. In addition, because the risk for hemorrhage is high among these patients, caution is also necessary when placing intravenous and other lines. For patients who have Lassa fever, Bolivian hemorrhagic fever, Congo-Crimean hemorrhagic fever, or Rift Valley fever, the antiviral agent ribavirin may offer some benefit [49].

Botulism

History and significance

Botulism is a syndrome caused by exposure to one or more of the seven neurotoxins produced by the bacillus *Clostridium botulinum*. The botulinum toxins are among the most potent toxins in existence. They are 100,000 times more toxic per microgram than the nerve agent sarin, which was used by the cult Aum Shinri Kyo in their terrorist attack in the Tokyo subway system in 1995. Theoretically, enough toxin is present in a single gram of crystallized botulinum toxin to kill more than 1 million people.

Most cases of naturally occurring botulism result from the ingestion of improperly prepared or canned foods; the disease is also associated, although rarely, with infected wounds or abscesses related to injection drug use. Terrorists could conceivably contaminate food supplies with the botulinum toxins or initiate a large-scale attack by dispersing the toxins through aerosol over a vast area [51]. Despite efforts to produce an effective botulinum toxin weapon, botulism is unlikely to ever be effectively deployed as a weapon of mass destruction. Aerosol delivery would require large quantities of toxin at the optimal time, because botulinum toxin quickly degrades in the environment and is rendered nonlethal within minutes after release. Municipal water reservoirs are most likely safe from contamination by terrorists, because ton quantities of toxin would be necessary due to the effects of dilution. Botulinum toxin is not stable for extended periods in water, and chlorination provides an effective means of destruction.

Clinical presentation

Unlike most other bioterrorism-related illness, botulism has a fairly characteristic presentation and therefore can usually be diagnosed from the clinical signs and symptoms alone. The clinical syndrome is similar regardless of whether the botulinum toxins are ingested or inhaled. Once absorbed, the toxins block the cholinergic synapses and thereby interfere with neurotransmission. After an incubation period of 1 to 5 days, patients generally present with neurologic manifestations. Bulbar palsies are extremely common, with ocular signs such as diplopia and mydriasis. Other bulbar effects may include dysarthria and dysphagia. Eventually, patients will experience progressive weakness, followed by skeletal muscle paralysis. The cause of death is usually respiratory failure. On physical examination, infected patients are generally afebrile, alert, and oriented. They may have postural hypotension, and some complain of dry mouth.

Diagnosis

Laboratory testing is generally not helpful. The diagnosis usually must be made on clinical and epidemiologic grounds. Botulinum toxins are generally difficult to detect, and most patients do not have antibody responses because the amount of toxin required to produce clinical symptoms is so small. Some bioassay tests are available, such as a mouse bioassay, in which the specimen is injected into mice that are then observed for changes. These assays are labor-intensive and take several days, and are only available in a few laboratories.

Infection control precautions

Standard universal procedures should be taken whenever a patient presents with botulism. Patients who may have the toxin on their skin as a result of aerosol exposure should bathe thoroughly with soap and water and discard their clothes.

Treatment and prophylaxis

The mainstay of treatment is hemodynamic and ventilatory support. Most patients who have botulism will survive if they are given proper ventilatory assistance. Full recovery, however, generally takes several weeks or months, during which the patient is required to remain on a ventilator, because new synapses must grow to replace the ones damaged by the botulinum toxin. Unfortunately, this strategy would present insurmountable logistical problems in the event of a terrorist attack, when hundreds or thousands of people may be afflicted with respiratory failure. Mechanical ventilators will be in short supply, and bag-ventilation would be impractical for weeks to months. The sudden demand for limited resources could make proper care for the many victims nearly impossible.

A trivalent equine botulinum antitoxin is available from the CDC and some state health departments [52]. Unfortunately, it is effective only in preventing further deterioration; it will not reverse muscle weakness that has already developed. It would not be available in adequate amounts to treat the number of people resulting from a large-scale exposure. Because the antitoxin is a horse serum product, skin testing for horse serum sensitivity is recommended before the drug is administered. A newer human botulism immunoglobulin has been shown to be effective for infant botulism [53], and would probably also be effective for preventing progression of botulism related to bioterrorism events.

Tularemia

History and significance

Otherwise known as *rabbit* or *deer fly fever*, tularemia is usually contracted after contact with infected animals or from the bites of infected deerflies, mosquitoes, or ticks. It can also be caused by the ingestion of contaminated food and water and the inhalation of contaminated air. The causative organism, *Francisella tularensis*, is a small, intracellular gram-negative coccobacillus. *F tularensis* remains viable for weeks in water, soil, carcasses, and hides, and for years in frozen meat. It is easily killed by heat and disinfectants but can survive for months in temperatures of freezing and below.

F tularensis was weaponized by the United States in the 1950s and 1960s during the offensive biowarfare program, and other countries are also suspected to have weaponized the organism. *F tularensis* could potentially be stabilized for weaponization and produced in either a wet or dried form for delivery in a terrorist attack [54]. As few as 10 to 50 organisms may cause disease if inhaled or injected intradermally; however, approximately 10^8 organisms are required to cause infection after oral ingestion.

Clinical presentation

Tularemia can manifest in several ways, depending on the route of infection. Ulceroglandular tularemia resulting from contact with infected animals is the most common form, accounting for up to 85% of cases. This form manifests as fever, chills, headache, malaise, an ulcerated skin lesion, and painful regional lymphadenopathy. Skin ulcers typically begin in the area of exposure to the organism, most commonly on the hands.

Typhoidal tularemia, which is caused by infectious aerosols, is the form most likely to appear after a terrorist attack. After an incubation period of 2 to 10 days, most victims present with fever, headache, chills, myalgia, nausea, vomiting, and diarrhea. They may also have cough and other respiratory symptoms. Initial laboratory evaluations are generally nonspecific. Approximately 80% of patients will have pneumonia. These nonspecific signs and symptoms would make a specific diagnosis of tularemia difficult in the event of a terrorist attack, leading to increased mortality. Case fatality rates of untreated naturally acquired typhoidal cases is approximately 35%, compared with 1% to 3% for appropriately treated cases.

Diagnosis

Tularemia can be diagnosed through culturing the organism from blood, ulcers, conjunctival exudates, sputum, gastric washings, and pharyngeal exudates, although culture is difficult and the yield is low. The organism grows poorly on standard media but can be grown on media containing cysteine or other sulfhydryl compounds (eg, glucose cysteine blood agar, thioglycollate broth). The laboratory should be notified if tularemia is suspected, because the organism represents a hazard to laboratory personnel. Culture should only be attempted using biosafety level 3 precautions.

Tularemia is usually diagnosed serologically using bacterial agglutination or ELISA. Antibodies to *F tularensis* appear within the first week of infection, but levels adequate to allow confidence in the specificity of the serologic diagnosis (titer > 1:160) do not appear until more than 2 weeks after infection [55]. Cross-reactions can occur with other organisms, such as

Brucella, Proteus, and *Yersinia.* Because antibodies may persist for years after infection, serologic diagnosis depends on a fourfold or greater increase in the tularemia tube agglutination or microagglutination titer during the course of the illness. Titers are usually negative during the first week of infection, become positive during the second week in 50% to 70% of cases, and achieve a maximum level in 4 to 8 weeks [56].

Infection control precautions

Although person-to-person transmission of tularemia is rare, health care personnel should follow standard universal precautions whenever managing patients who have the disease.

Treatment and prophylaxis

The traditional treatment for patients who have tularemia is a 10- to 14-day course of streptomycin, but this agent may not be readily available in the event of an attack. Other agents that have proven effective against the disease include gentamicin, tetracycline, chloramphenicol, and fluoroquinolones [57]. Ciprofloxacin or doxycycline could be used for postexposure protection against tularemia, based on in vitro susceptibilities. A 2-week course should be effective as postexposure prophylaxis when given within 24 hours of aerosol exposure.

Category B agents

Coxiella burnetii *(Q fever)*

History and significance

Not all potential agents of bioterrorism cause fulminant, life-threatening illnesses; some produce milder, longer-lasting illnesses. Q fever is a good example of the latter. The disease has a long incubation period, after which it tends to produce nonspecific, fairly mild symptoms. Only very rarely is it fatal. However, a terrorist group could still disrupt and terrify a community by causing nonfatal illness.

Q fever is an acute or chronic zoonotic illness caused by the rickettsial organism *Coxiella burnetii.* The illness was described during a 1935 outbreak in Queensland, Australia, and was called Q (query) fever because the origin was not currently identified.

Q fever occurs worldwide and usually results from exposure to infected livestock such as sheep, cattle, or goats. Infected animals are usually asymptomatic; parturient animals may have large numbers of organisms present in the placenta, resulting in environmental contamination. Humans typically become infected through inhaling aerosols containing *C burnetii.* The organism proliferates in the lung and then spreads through the bloodstream.

C burnetii has a spore-like form that can survive for weeks or months in the environment. The organism can survive heat and drying and can be disseminated through airborne spread. *C burnetii* is highly infectious to humans; a single viable organism is adequate to cause infection. Because of these characteristics, it is considered suitable for use as a bioweapon.

Clinical presentation

The presenting symptoms of Q fever are nonspecific. In fact, many infections appear to be asymptomatic. In those who become ill, the most common findings are fever, chills, and headache. Onset may be sudden or gradual, and the incubation period can vary considerably from approximately 10 days up to several weeks. Most patients have a self-limited febrile illness that resolves within 1 or 2 weeks. Overall mortality is low: 2.4% in one large series of hospitalized patients [58]. However, many patients report malaise and fatigue that persist for months.

Q fever may manifest as pneumonia. Many patients who have Q fever have radiographic evidence of pneumonia but no cough. If cough is present, it is usually nonproductive. Severe headache is frequently associated with Q fever pneumonia. Hepatic transaminase levels are frequently elevated, but the peripheral white blood cell count is usually normal. Some patients have a rapidly progressing pneumonia syndrome similar to Legionnaire's disease. Although Q fever pneumonia may have various radiographic appearances, multiple rounded opacities (often pleural-based) are a suggestive pattern. Pleural effusion (usually small) is found in approximately one third of cases [59].

Q fever can also have various chronic manifestations, including endocarditis, intravascular infection, hepatitis, and osteomyelitis. Endocarditis typically involves abnormal or prosthetic valves but can sometimes develop in normal valves. *C burnetii* will not grow in routine blood cultures, so culture-negative endocarditis is a typical clinical picture. Liver involvement may manifest as acute hepatitis or as a fever of unknown origin, with granulomas found on liver biopsy.

Diagnosis

Most laboratories do not have the facilities to isolate *C burnetii*. Serologic testing through complement fixation, indirect fluorescent antibody (IFA) or ELISA is the mainstay of diagnosis for Q fever. However, titers may not be elevated until 2 to 3 weeks into the illness. Convalescent titers characteristically show a fourfold increase 2 or 3 months after onset of illness.

Infection control precautions

Human-to-human spread of Q fever does not seem to occur, and therefore isolation is not required. However, tissues from patients who have Q fever may pose a threat to laboratory workers and should be processed under biosafety level 3 conditions.

Treatment and prophylaxis

Several antibiotics have activity against *C burnetii* and seem to shorten the duration of illness. Antibiotics also seem to prevent illness when given during the incubation period [60]. Tetracyclines are most commonly used for treatment. Other drugs that have been used include macrolides, quinolones, chloramphenicol, rifampin, and trimethoprim-sulfamethoxazole. The optimal duration of therapy is unclear. Treatment for uncomplicated infections or prophylaxis is generally given for 5 to 7 days. Prolonged combination treatment (eg, doxycycline plus a quinolone or rifampin) is usually given for chronic infection such as endocarditis. A vaccine against Q fever is being used in Australia but is not licensed in the United States [61].

Brucella *species (brucellosis)*

History and significance

Brucellosis is a zoonotic infection that can have various manifestations in humans. *Brucella* species are small, aerobic, slow-growing gram-negative coccobacilli. The genus *Brucella* is divided into several species on the basis of preferred animal hosts and other features. The main manifestations in animals are abortion and sterility. Humans can become infected from (1) direct contact with animal secretions through breaks in the skin, (2) infected aerosols, or (3) ingestion of unpasteurized dairy products. Brucellae are facultative intracellular pathogens, and replication and spread seem to occur through lymphatics and hematogenous dissemination. *Brucella* species can survive for many weeks in soil or water. *B suis* was weaponized by the United States in the 1940s and 1950s; other countries are also suspected to have weaponized brucellae. Brucella organisms are highly infectious when aerosolized; consequently, inhalation will be the most likely route of infection during a terrorist attack. The organism could be spread as a slurry in bomblets or as a dry aerosol [61].

Clinical presentation

Clinical symptoms of brucellosis are varied and nonspecific. Like Q fever, brucellosis can begin insidiously, with an influenza-like illness. Symptoms generally begin 2 to 4 weeks after exposure, but the incubation period can be 8 weeks or more. The infection tends to localize in tissues with large numbers of macrophages, such as lung, spleen, liver, central nervous system (CNS), bone marrow, and synovium. Symptoms vary because of the widespread nature of infection. In most instances, the intermittent fever phase lasts for several weeks, followed by a period of remission, during which symptoms may wane or disappear altogether. The fever and other symptoms then recur. This pattern of periodic febrile waves and remission can last for months or even years. Although chronic cases of brucellosis can be very debilitating, the disease is rarely fatal. Fever, chills, sweats, anorexia, headache, and malaise are common manifestations. Although patients may complain of many symptoms, physical findings are often lacking.

Liver involvement is common, although transaminase levels are usually only mildly elevated. Hepatic granulomas are characteristic of some species, such as *B abortus*. Several skeletal complications are also found, including arthritis, osteomyelitis, and tenosynovitis. Large weight-bearing joints (eg, sacroiliac, hips, knees, ankles) are most commonly involved. Hematologic findings include anemia, leukopenia, and thrombocytopenia. The rare serious complications of brucellosis include endocarditis and CNS infection. Although depression and difficulty concentrating are common complaints in patients who have brucellosis, direct invasion of the CNS (eg, meningitis, encephalitis) occurs in fewer than 5% of infected individuals [62]. Endocarditis occurs in fewer than 2% of cases but is responsible for most deaths.

Diagnosis

Brucellosis can be diagnosed through isolation of the organism in cultures or by serology. Because brucellae are slow-growing, the laboratory should be alerted to hold culture specimens for at least 4 weeks if brucellosis is suspected. Cultures of bone marrow have a higher yield than blood. Rapid bacterial identification systems used by many laboratories may reduce the time to isolation, but misidentification of brucellae with these systems has been reported [63]. A presumptive diagnosis can be made on the basis of high or rising antibody titers. Most patients who have infection have titers higher than 1:160. Febrile agglutinin tests are not adequately sensitive. PCR techniques may soon yield a rapid method of diagnosing brucellosis.

Infection control precautions

Because human-to-human transmission seems to be rare, isolation is not necessary. However, the organisms are highly infectious through aerosol, and culture specimens may pose a threat to laboratory workers. The laboratory should be notified if brucellosis is suspected; laboratory biosafety level 2 or 3 precautions are recommended. Contact isolation should be used for patients who have open draining lesions.

Treatment and prophylaxis

Although most patients will recover without treatment, antibiotics reduce the severity and duration of illness. Many antibiotics have in vitro activity, but those with good intracellular penetration are most effective clinically. Combination treatment is most effective. Doxycycline plus rifampin for 6 weeks is the most commonly used regimen. Gentamicin or streptomycin is sometimes included in the regimen for more severe infections such as endocarditis. No effective human vaccine is available for brucellosis.

Antibiotics will unlikely prevent disease if given before the onset of symptoms, although the optimal regimen is unknown. Because of the long incubation period, the opportunity for prophylaxis is greater with brucellosis than for some other agents with shorter incubation periods, such as anthrax or tularemia. An economic model estimated that the economic impact of a bioterrorist attack with brucellosis on a population of 100,000 people would be approximately $478 million. Timely intervention with antibiotic prophylaxis could reduce the economic impact through preventing illness [64].

Burkholderia mallei *(glanders)*

History and significance

Glanders is a disease of horses, mules, and donkeys caused by the bacterium *Burkholderia mallei* (previously known as *Pseudomonas mallei*). The infection can also occur in humans and other animals. Human infection is rare but can be severe. *B mallei* is a nonmotile, gram-negative bacillus. The route of naturally occurring infection is unclear, but infection is believed to occur through broken skin or nasal mucosa contaminated with infected material. Infection also seems to occur through an aerosol route, as evidenced by infections in laboratory workers from routine handling of cultures [65,66]. Its ability to cause serious illness and infect through aerosol indicate that *B mallei* may have potential use in bioterrorism. In fact, this organism has been used as a bioweapon; animals were deliberately infected with glanders during World War I [67].

Melioidosis is a human illness caused by *B pseudomallei*, which is clinically similar to glanders but does not seem to be particularly infectious through aerosol.

Clinical presentation

Infection from inoculation through a break in the skin typically results in a tender nodule with local lymphangitis. Inoculation of the eyes, nose, and mouth can result in mucopurulent discharge with ulcerating granulomas. With systemic invasion, a generalized papular or pustular eruption is frequent. This septicemic form is often fatal within 7 to 10 days. The incubation period after infection through inhalation (most likely in a bioterrorism event) is approximately 10 to 14 days. The most common manifestations include fever, myalgias, headache, and pleuritic chest pain. Lymphadenopathy or splenomegaly may be present. The disease often manifests as pneumonia [65].

Diagnosis

The organism can be difficult to identify. Blood cultures are usually negative, except in the terminal stages of septicemia. Automated bacterial identification systems used in many laboratories may not correctly identify *B mallei*. Serologic tests will usually show a rise in titers by the second week, but agglutination titers are not very specific. Complement fixation titers are more specific but less sensitive. Serologic tests are not standardized or widely available. *B mallei* and *B pseudomallei* cannot be distinguished morphologically, but a PCR procedure has been developed that can differentiate the two [68].

Infection control precautions

Because person-to-person transmission can occur, isolation is indicated. Culture specimens pose a threat to laboratory personnel, and therefore the laboratory should be notified if *B mallei* is suspected. Biosafety level 3 precautions are indicated.

Treatment and prophylaxis

The paucity of human cases has prevented any systematic study of treatment. Sulfadiazine has been effective in experimental animal infections and humans. Agents known to be effective for human melioidosis include tetracyclines, trimethoprim- sulfamethoxazole, amoxicillin-clavulanate, and chloramphenicol. In vitro, *B mallei* is susceptible to aminoglycosides, macrolides, quinolones, doxycycline, piperacillin, ceftazidime, and imipenem [69]. No vaccine is available.

Alphaviruses

History and significance

Venezuelan Equine Encephalomyelitis and Eastern and Western Equine Encephalomyelitis (VEE, EEE, and WEE, respectively) are mosquito-borne viral infections found in North and South America. EEE occurs primarily along the eastern and gulf coasts of the United States. Although human illness is rare, the case-fatality rate can be as high as 50% to 70%. WEE viruses are found primarily west of the Mississippi. During an epidemic, WEE infection rates are much higher than for EEE, but the case fatality rate is much lower (approximately 3%–4%). Outbreaks occur primarily in the summer, and equine cases greatly outnumber human cases. VEE occurs in many areas of South and Central America, and outbreaks have occurred in North America.

These alphaviruses are limited in their geographic distribution by the mosquito vector, and therefore finding these viruses outside the endemic areas should arouse suspicion of an intentional release. All of these viruses are highly infectious through aerosol. Because they are stable during storage and can be produced in large amounts with unsophisticated equipment, they are regarded as having potential for weaponization [61].

Clinical presentation

Most infections with these viruses result in nonspecific symptoms of fever, headache, and myalgia. Only a fraction of individuals infected will experience progression to frank encephalitis. Viral encephalitides should be included in the differential diagnosis of nonspecific viral syndromes after a possible bioterrorism event. Reports of ill horses in the vicinity would obviously suggest an equine encephalitis virus. Whether aerosol exposure, as in a bioterrorism event, would lead to a pattern of symptoms different from that of the mosquito-borne illness is unknown.

EEE is the most severe of these infections, with high mortality rates and high rates of neurologic sequelae [70]. WEE and VEE have lower rates of progression to neurologic symptoms. Infants and elderly individuals are more prone to developing encephalitis. In people who develop encephalitis, the initial viral prodrome is followed by confusion and somnolence, which may progress to coma. Peripheral blood counts often show leukopenia in the early stages of illness, which can progress to leukocytosis. CSF protein is elevated, and lymphocytic pleocytosis is usually present.

Diagnosis

Virus can sometimes be isolated from blood during the early stages of illness, but viremia has usually resolved by the time symptoms of encephalitis develop. Virus can sometimes be isolated from CSF or postmortem brain tissue. The specific viral pathogen is generally identified through serologic testing of the CSF or serum (or both), but these results will not be available until later. Virus-specific IgM antibodies can be detected with ELISA [71]. Subsequent testing of convalescent serum may confirm the diagnosis but will not be helpful in initial management. Physicians should attempt to obtain enough CSF for specialized testing if encephalitis is a diagnostic possibility. Experimental PCR assays have been developed for several viral pathogens and will likely become more standardized and readily available in the future.

Infection control precautions

Isolation is not necessary since person-to-person transmission does not occur.

Treatment and prophylaxis

No specific treatment for these viral encephalitides. Treatment is supportive. Inactivated vaccines are available for EEE, WEE, and VEE, but none is widely used because of problems with poor immunogenicity and need for multiple doses. A live attenuated vaccine is available for VEE but has a high incidence of side effects, such as fever, headache, and malaise. Newer vaccines using recombinant technology are in development.

Ricin toxin from ricinus communis (castor beans)

History and significance

Ricin is a protein toxin derived from the castor bean plant. Castor beans are easily obtained worldwide, and it is relatively easy to extract the toxin. One million tons of castor beans are processed annually in the production of castor oil worldwide; the waste mash from this process is approximately 5% ricin by weight. Ricin was used in the assassination of Bulgarian exile Georgi Markov in London in 1978. Markov was attacked with a specially engineered weapon disguised as an umbrella, which implanted a ricin-containing pellet into his leg [72].

Ricin toxin is somewhat less toxic by weight compared with botulinum toxin or staphylococcal enterotoxin B, but can be produced in large quantities easily. Ricin toxin is stable and can be disseminated as an aerosol. It is toxic through several routes of exposure, including respiratory and gastrointestinal.

Clinical presentation

Ricin toxin inhibits protein synthesis. When inhaled as an aerosol, the toxin can produce symptoms within 4 to 8 hours. Typical symptoms include fever, chest tightness, cough, dyspnea, nausea, arthralgias, and profuse sweating. With a sublethal dose of toxin, the symptoms should improve within several hours. In animal studies, lethal doses produced necrosis of the respiratory tract and alveolar filling in 36 to 72 hours after exposure.

When ingested, ricin causes severe gastrointestinal symptoms, such as nausea, vomiting, and diarrhea. With large toxin exposures, this may be associated with gastrointestinal hemorrhage and hepatic, splenic, and renal necrosis. Death can occur from hypovolemic shock [73]. Ricin toxin may also cause disseminated intravascular coagulation, microcirculatory failure, and multiple organ failure if given intravenously in laboratory animals.

Diagnosis

Diagnosis of ricin poisoning would be primarily clinical and epidemiologic. ELISA testing can be performed on serum, but this modality would not be widely available in most laboratories [74]. Acute and convalescent sera could be obtained from survivors to measure antibody response for diagnostic confirmation.

Infection control precautions

This toxin-mediated syndrome has no potential for person-to-person spread. Patients who are grossly contaminated may need to change their clothes and wash with soap and water.

Treatment and prophylaxis

Treatment of ricin poisoning is supportive. Respiratory support may be needed for pulmonary edema. Gastric decontamination with charcoal may have some benefit for ingestions. Fluids may be required to replace gastrointestinal losses. Vaccines against ricin toxin are currently under development [75].

Epsilon toxin of Clostridium perfringens

History and significance

Clostridium perfringens is an anaerobic, gram-positive, spore-forming bacillus. This ubiquitous organism is present in soil throughout the world and has been found in the stool of virtually every vertebrate organism ever tested [76]. Clostridium species can produce various toxins, and these are responsible for illness. Enterotoxin-producing strains of C perfringens type A cause a mild form of food poisoning that is common worldwide. Large amounts of this toxin could be produced for intentional exposure.

Clinical presentation

Within hours of exposure, gastrointestinal symptoms such as watery diarrhea, nausea, and abdominal cramps will develop. Fever is rare. Spontaneous resolution typically occurs within a day, and fatalities are rare. The *C perfringens* enterotoxin can act as a superantigen and is a potent stimulator of human lymphocytes. Large exposure through aerosol or ingestion could lead to more severe systemic symptoms.

Diagnosis

Enterotoxin can be detected in stool with latex agglutination or ELISA, but these tests are not widely available. Cultures are not of value because *C perfringens* is normally found in stool.

Infection control precautions

Because this is a toxin-mediated syndrome, no potential exists for person-to-person spread.

Treatment and prophylaxis

Treatment is supportive.

Staphylococcus enterotoxin B

History and significance

Staphylococcal enterotoxin B (SEB) is a common cause of food poisoning caused by a heat-stable toxin produced by the ubiquitous organism *Staphylococcus aureus*. The toxin is relatively stable in aerosols (more stable than botulinum toxin); even low doses can cause symptoms when inhaled. Although rarely fatal, a high percentage of those exposed could become seriously ill within a few hours. It could also be used to contaminate food or water supplies.

Clinical presentation

SEB is a potent activator of T cells, and most of the clinical manifestations are mediated by the patient's own immune system. Symptoms begin 3 to 12 hours after exposure. Typical symptoms are high fever, headache, myalgia, prostration, and dry cough. Vomiting and diarrhea may result from swallowed toxin. Patients may be incapacitated for up to 2 weeks. In severe cases, pulmonary edema or adult respiratory distress syndrome may develop. In rare cases, death occurs from dehydration.

Diagnosis

The diagnosis of SEB intoxication is primarily clinical and epidemiologic. Practically speaking, a specific diagnosis of SEB would be very difficult. The symptoms are nonspecific and overlap with many other clinical syndromes, including those of other bioterrorism agents. Because of the short incubation period, this agent is more likely to cause a sudden cluster of cases in a localized area compared with many other bioterrorism agents. The toxin may be identified with ELISA of nasal swabs after aerosol exposure, or the antigen can be detected in urine [61]. Neither of these tests is readily available.

Infection control precautions

Because this is a toxin-mediated syndrome, no potential exists for person-to-person spread. However, if patients are grossly contaminated after a recent exposure, health care workers could be exposed to the toxin on skin or clothing. A simple change of clothes and shower with soap and water would provide adequate decontamination.

Treatment and prophylaxis

Treatment is supportive. Some patients may require rehydration for fluid losses, although care must be taken to avoid pulmonary edema in more severe intoxications. Ventilatory support may be required in severe cases. Vaccines are under development.

Food-borne and waterborne pathogens

History and significance

Although most agents considered more likely to be used for bioterrorism would be disseminated through aerosol, food- or waterborne agents could be used. In fact, Shigella and Salmonella have already been used in intentional exposures in the United States. Shigella was used to contaminate donuts given to fellow workers by a disgruntled employee and caused 12 cases of diarrhea [77]. Salmonella was used by a religious commune in Oregon to contaminate local salad bars, leading to more than 750 cases of gastroenteritis [78].

Food- and waterborne agents would be less likely than airborne agents to be involved in a large-scale attack, because it is more difficult to expose large numbers of people. Standard treatment of municipal water supplies would preclude survival of most biologic agents and inactivates most biological toxins. Food-borne outbreaks are generally limited to small groups of people. However, more centralized processing of foods for mass marketing may increase the potential for widespread food-borne outbreaks, as has been shown by multistate outbreaks of Listeria and Salmonella resulting from contamination in food-processing facilities [79,80].

Salmonella species, Shigella dysenteriae, Escherichia coli O157:H7, and Vibrio cholerae are all bacterial causes of food-borne gastroenteritis. Salmonella, Shigella, and E coli all cause illness sporadically in the United States [81]. Cholera is a cause of severe gastroenteritis in developing countries but is only occasionally imported into the United States.

Cryptosporidium parvum is a protozoal organism that is also associated with diarrhea. C parvum can be spread by contamination of food or water and has been involved in outbreaks related to swimming pools. Because it is resistant to chlorine, *C parvum* can survive in swimming pools and municipal water supplies. *C parvum* was associated with a massive outbreak caused by contamination of the municipal water supply in Milwaukee, Wisconsin, in 1993 [82]. More than 400,000 people became ill, resulting in more than 40,000 health care visits and 4000 hospitalizations.

Clinical presentation

These infections generally present with diarrhea, sometimes associated with nausea, vomiting, fever, and abdominal cramps. The incubation period is approximately 1 to 3 days. Gastroenteritis caused by *Shigella* is often associated with blood or mucus in the stool. *Salmonella typhi* and *S paratyphi* can produce a typhoidal syndrome, with gradual onset of fever, headache, malaise, myalgias, and constipation. Diarrhea is uncommon. Cholera is associated with severe watery diarrhea, which can cause death from dehydration within hours.

E coli O157:H7 is notable for being associated with bloody diarrhea, but Salmonella or Shigella can also be associated with this condition [83]. *E coli* O157:H7 produces a Shiga toxin associated with development of hemolytic uremic syndrome (HUS) [84]. HUS is characterized by hemolytic anemia, thrombocytopenia, and renal insufficiency. Approximately 6% of people with bloody diarrhea caused by *E coli* O157:H7 will develop HUS, but the rate is higher (about 10%) in children younger than 10 years. The mortality rate associated with HUS is 3% to 5%.

C parvum typically causes watery diarrhea associated with crampy abdominal pain. The incubation period is usually approximately a week but can sometimes extend up to several weeks. Illness can sometimes last for many weeks.

Diagnosis

Routine stool cultures for enteropathogens will identify agents such as *Salmonella* and *Shigella*. Many laboratories do not routinely test for *E coli* O157:H7 and other Shiga toxin–producing strains of *E coli*, so the laboratory should be notified if this agent is suspected (eg, afebrile patient with bloody diarrhea). *E coli* O157:H7 appears as a colorless colony on sorbitol MacConkey agar. These colonies can be tested for O157 antigen using a commercial kit. Stool cultures can also be tested directly for Shiga toxin using a commercial kit. *V cholerae* requires special media to grow, so the laboratory should be notified if cholera is suspected. *C parvum* can be identified with a modified acid-fast stain of stool or with fluorescent stain.

Infection control precautions

Standard body fluid precautions should prevent spread of these organisms. Patients should be instructed to be extra vigilant about handwashing after using the bathroom.

Treatment and prophylaxis

Treatment of these infections is generally supportive. Most infections with *Salmonella* and *Shigella* are self-limited and will resolve without specific treatment within a few days. Antimicrobial treatment may reduce the duration and severity of symptoms. *Salmonella* is susceptible to quinolones, azithromycin, and third-generation cephalosporins. Resistance to trimethoprim-sulfamethoxazole seems to be increasing, and antimicrobial-resistant organisms seem likely to be used in a bioterrorism event. *Shigella* is susceptible to fluoroquinolones, trimethoprim-sulfamethoxazole, and azithromycin. *E coli* O157:H7 infection should not be treated with antimicrobials or antimotility agents, because treatment may increase toxin production and thereby increase the risk for hemolytic uremic syndrome. Treatment of cholera typically requires large amounts of intravenous fluids and replacement of electrolytes. Oral administration of ciprofloxacin or doxycycline is effective for cholera. No antimicrobial agent has proven efficacy for *C parvum* infection, although paromomycin and azithromycin have been used in patients who have AIDS experiencing chronic diarrhea caused by this organism.

Category C agents

Nipah virus

History and significance

In April 1999, an outbreak of 257 cases of encephalitis (100 fatal) was reported in Malaysia [85]. A previously unrecognized paramyxovirus called *Nipah* was identified as the cause. Pigs appeared to be the primary source of human infection in this outbreak.

Clinical presentation

Patients in the reported outbreak presented with fever, headache, and myalgias and eventually developed signs of meningitis or encephalitis. A few patients had respiratory symptoms.

Diagnosis

Identification of Nipah virus requires specialized testing in a reference laboratory, such as the CDC or USAMRIID. IgM antibodies can be detected in blood and CSF. Better diagnostic tests for this recently discovered agent are under development [86].

Infection control precautions

Person-to-person spread of Nipah virus has not been identified. However, virus has been isolated from respiratory secretions and urine of patients infected with Nipah virus [87]. Pending further study of the potential for person-to-person spread, strict isolation would be prudent for patients suspected of being infected with this virus.

Treatment and prophylaxis

Treatment is primarily supportive. A small, open-label trial conducted during the outbreak in Malaysia showed a 36% reduction of mortality among patients who had acute Nipah virus encephalitis with ribavirin [88].

Hantaviruses

History and significance

Hantaviruses are in the family Bunyaviridae, which also comprises California encephalitis virus and several hemorrhagic fever viruses. Hantaviruses are found in many rodent species worldwide. Hantavirus and several related viruses cause a syndrome of fever, thrombocytopenia, and renal insufficiency; the disease occurs primarily in Eastern Asia. Sin nombre virus (SNV), a similar virus, was identified as the cause of several cases of severe pulmonary edema and shock (hantavirus pulmonary syndrome) in the southwestern United States in 1993 [89]. Aerosols of virus-contaminated rodent urine or feces seemed to be the mechanism of transmission in these cases. Because aerosol transmission is possible, the virus is believed to have potential for weaponization.

Clinical presentation

Hantavirus pulmonary syndrome (HPS) begins with a viral prodrome of fever and myalgias. Respiratory symptoms, including cough and dyspnea, begin after several days. Laboratory investigations may reveal an elevated hematocrit, leukocytosis, mild thrombocytopenia, and elevated liver transaminases. In severe cases, the illness progresses to pulmonary edema, with respiratory failure and shock [90].

Diagnosis

Hantaviruses are difficult to isolate in viral culture. In the acute phase of the disease, the clinical diagnosis may be confirmed through serology or PCR. ELISA and IFA are available to identify antibody to hantaviruses [91]. An immunoblot assay is also available.

Infection control precautions

Person-to-person transmission of naturally occurring SNV in the United States has not been identified. However, it has been identified in Argentina, including a fatal infection in a physician who also transmitted the virus to his family [92,93]. Because of the potential for person-to-person spread of a virus used in an intentional attack, using respiratory isolation would be prudent for persons who have suspected HPS related to a bioterrorism event.

Treatment and prophylaxis

Treatment of HPS is primarily supportive. Extracorporeal membrane oxygenation has been used in severe cases [94]. An open-label trial of ribavirin for HPS failed to show any benefit. Controlled trials of ribavirin are ongoing. Vaccines are under development.

Other agents

Several arthropod-borne viruses might have potential for use as bioweapons, including the flaviviruses that cause yellow fever and tick-borne encephalitis. Person-to-person transmission of flaviviruses does not appear to occur, except through the arthropod vectors.

Yellow fever is a mosquito-borne virus of historical interest because of large outbreaks that played a role in development of the Americas. The disease has been greatly diminished through mosquito control and vaccination, although sporadic outbreaks still occur. The severity of illness can range from a mild self-limited viral syndrome to a fatal hemorrhagic fever [95]. After an incubation period of several days, symptoms begin as fever, headache, and myalgias. Conjunctivitis, relative bradycardia, and leukopenia may be present. Jaundice occurs secondary to hepatitis, and gastrointestinal bleeding may also occur. Death can occur 7 to 10 days after onset. Treatment of yellow fever is supportive. The illness is preventable with the attenuated 17D vaccine, which produces immunity in approximately 95% of those vaccinated.

Tick-borne encephalitis occurs in many areas of Europe and Asia. Infection can also occur from consumption of unpasteurized milk products. Most infections are asymptomatic or only mildly symptomatic, but a small fraction of infected individuals can develop encephalitis. Only approximately 1% of encephalitis cases are fatal, mostly in elderly individuals [96]. No specific therapy exists for flavivirus encephalitis.

Multidrug-resistant tuberculosis has become a significant problem in many areas of the world over the past several decades. Although illness progression and person-to-person transmission occur slowly, the ability to disseminate through aerosol and difficulty treating multidrug-resistant strains could make the organism attractive as a bioweapon. Treatment options for highly resistant strains are severely limited [97].

Summary

Various agents have potential for use as weapons of bioterrorism. Knowledge of the likely organisms may be useful in preparations to mitigate the effects of a bioterrorism event. Recognizing the clinical presentation of these organisms could help physicians identify infection quickly, allowing more appropriate management and possible prophylaxis of other individuals who may have been exposed. Although many of these agents do not have specific treatments, those that do are important to recognize. Which infections require isolation is also important to know because of potential for person-to-person spread.

If a bioterrorism event occurs, the expertise of emergency physicians and infectious disease specialists will be critical to mitigate the effects of the disaster. Emergency physicians will be on the front line when large numbers of ill and potentially contagious patients present for care. Infectious disease specialists will be essential in providing expertise for specialized diagnostic testing, identifying treatment options when resources may be limited, and advising on infection control and prophylaxis. Disaster planning for bioterrorism should incorporate consideration of surge capacity, infection control, and mobilization of resources for vaccination, antimicrobial treatment, and prophylaxis for large numbers of people.

References

[1] Keim M, Kaufmann AF. Principles for emergency response to bioterrorism. Ann Emerg Med 1999;34(2):177–82.

[2] Richards CF, Burstein JL, Waeckerle JF, et al. Emergency physicians and biological terrorism. Ann Emerg Med 1999;34(2):183–90.

[3] Tham KY. An emergency department response to severe acute respiratory syndrome: a prototype response to bioterrorism. Ann Emerg Med 2004;43(1):6–14.

[4] Macintyre AG, Christopher GW, Eitzen E, et al. Weapons of mass destruction events with contaminated casualties: effective planning for health care facilities. JAMA 2000;283(2): 242–9.

[5] Rubinson L, Nuzzo JB, Talmor DS, et al. Augmentation of hospital critical care capacity after bioterrorist attacks or epidemics. Crit Care Med 2005;33(10):2393–403.

[6] Wetter DC, Daniell WE, Treser CD. Hospital preparedness for victims of chemical or biological terrorism. Am J Public Health 2001;91(5):710–6.

[7] Centers for Disease Control and Prevention. Biological and chemical terrorism: strategic plan for preparedness and response. MMWR Recomm Rep 2000;49(RR04):1–14.

[8] Hupert N, Wattson D, Cuomo J, et al. Anticipating demand for emergency health services due to medication-related adverse events after rapid mass prophylaxis campaigns. Acad Emerg Med 2007;14(3):268–74.

[9] Rothman RE, Irvin CB, Moran GJ, et al. Respiratory hygiene in the emergency department. Ann Emerg Med 2006;48(5):570–82.

[10] Moran GJ, Fuchs MA, Jarvis WR, et al. Tuberculosis infection control practices in United States emergency departments. Ann Emerg Med 1995;26(3):283–9.

[11] Mead K, Johnson D. An evaluation of portable high-efficiency particulate air filtration for expedient patient isolation in epidemic and emergency response. Ann Emerg Med 2004; 44(6):635–45.

[12] Moran GJ, Kyriacou DN, Newdow MA, et al. Emergency department sentinel surveillance for emerging infectious diseases. Ann Emerg Med 1995;26(3):351–4.

[13] Moran GJ, Talan DA. CDC update commentary: public health surveillance for smallpox— United States, 2003–2005. Ann Emerg Med 2007;50(1):52–4.

[14] Moran GJ, Talan DA. CDC update commentary—syndromic surveillance for bioterrorism following the attacks on the world trade center—New York City, 2001. Ann Emerg Med 2003;41(3):417–8.

[15] U.S. Dept. of Health and Human Services. HIPAA. Available at: http://www.hhs.gov/ocr/hipaa/. Accessed December 7, 2007.

[16] Bourgeois FT, Olson KL, Brownstein JS, et al. Validation of syndromic surveillance for respiratory infections. Ann Emerg Med 2006;47(3):265–71.

[17] Christopher GW, Cieslak TJ, Pavlin JA, et al. Biological warfare, a historical perspective. JAMA 1997;278(5):412–7.

[18] Meselson M, Guillemin J, Hugh-Jones M, et al. The Sverdlovsk anthrax outbreak of 1979. Science 1994;266(5188):1202–8.

[19] Keim P, Smith KL, Keys C, et al. Molecular investigation of the Aum Shinrikyo anthrax release in Kameido, Japan. J Clin Microbiol 2001;39(12):4566–7.

[20] Bush L, Abrams B, Beall A, et al. Index case of fatal inhalational anthrax due to bioterrorism in the United States. N Engl J Med 2001;345(22):1607–10.

[21] Centers for Disease Control and Prevention. Investigation of bioterrorism-related anthrax, 2001. MMWR Morb Mortal Wkly Rep 2001;50(48):1008–10.

[22] Jernigan J, Stephens D, Ashford D, et al. Bioterrorism-related inhalational anthrax: the first 10 cases reported in the United States. Emerg Infect Dis 2001;7(6):933–44.

[23] Friedlander A. Anthrax. In: Sidell FR, Takafuji ET, Franz DR, editors. Textbook of military medicine: medical aspects of chemical and biological warfare. Washington, DC: TMM Publications; 1997. p. 467–78.

[24] Borio L, Frank D, Mani V, et al. Death due to bioterrorism-related inhalational anthrax: report of 2 patients. JAMA 2001;286(20):2554–9.

[25] Mayer T, Bersoff-Matcha S, Murphy C, et al. Clinical presentation of inhalational anthrax following bioterrorism exposure: report of 2 surviving patients. JAMA 2001;286(20): 2549–53.

[26] Centers for Disease Control and Prevention. Considerations for distinguishing influenza-like illness from inhalational anthrax. MMWR Morb Mortal Wkly Rep 2001;50(44):984–6.

[27] Holty JE, Kim RY, Bravata DM. Anthrax: a systematic review of atypical presentations. Ann Emerg Med 2006;48(2):200–11.

[28] Holty JE, Bravata DM, Liu H, et al. Systematic review: a century of inhalational anthrax cases from 1900 to 2005. Ann Intern Med 2006;144(4):270–80.

[29] Moran GJ. Commentary: bioterrorism alleging use of anthrax and interim guidelines for management. Ann Emerg Med 1999;34(2):229–32.

[30] Inglesby TV, Henderson DA, Bartlett JG, et al. Anthrax as a biological weapon: medical and public health management. JAMA 1999;281(18):1735–45.

[31] Kyriacou DN, Yarnold PR, Stein AC, et al. Discriminating inhalational anthrax from community-acquired pneumonia using chest radiograph findings and a clinical algorithm. Chest 2007;131(2):489–96.

[32] Dixon TC, Meselson M, Guillemin J, et al. Anthrax. N Engl J Med 1999;341(11):815–26.

[33] Inglesby TV, O'Toole T, Henderson DA, et al. Anthrax as a biological weapon, 2002: updated recommendations for management. JAMA 2002;287(17):2236–52.

[34] Friedlander AM, Pittman PR, Parker GW. Anthrax vaccine. JAMA 1999;282(22):2104–6.

[35] CDC. Surveillance for adverse events associated with anthrax vaccination—U.S. Dept. of Defense, 1998–2000. MMWR Morb Mortal Wkly Rep 2000;49(16):341–5.

[36] Darling RG, Catlett CL, Huebner KD, et al. Threats in bioterrorism. I: CDC category A agents. Emerg Med Clin North Am 2002;20(2):273–309.

[37] Willman D. New anthrax vaccine doomed by lobbying; America's sole supplier faced oblivion if its rival's product was adopted. It was time to call on its connections. Los Angeles Times. December 2, 2007;Part A:A1.

[38] Alibek K. Biohazard. New York: Random House; 1999.

[39] Inglesby TV, Dennis DT, Henderson DA, et al. Plague as a biological weapon. JAMA 2000; 283(17):2281–90.

[40] Henderson DA, Inglesby TV, Bartlett JG, et al. Smallpox as a biological weapon: medical and public health management. JAMA 1999;281(22):2127–37.

[41] Henderson DA. Smallpox: clinical and epidemiologic features. Emerg Infect Dis 1999;5(4): 537–9.

[42] Bartlett J, Borio L, Radonovich L, et al. Smallpox vaccination in 2003: key information for clinicians. Clin Infect Dis 2003;36(7):883–902.

[43] Centers for Disease Control and Prevention. Update: adverse events following civilian smallpox vaccination—United States, 2003. MMWR Morb Mortal Wkly Rep 2004;53(05):106–7.

[44] Centers for Disease Control and Prevention. Vulvar vaccinia infection after sexual contact with a military smallpox vaccinee—Alaska, 2006. MMWR Morb Mortal Wkly Rep 2007; 56(17):417–9.

[45] Kwon N, Raven MC, Chiang WK, et al. Emergency physicians' perspectives on smallpox vaccination. Acad Emerg Med 2003;10(6):599–605.

[46] Moran GJ, Everett WW, Karras DJ, et al. Smallpox vaccination for emergency physicians: joint statement of the AAEM and SAEM. J Emerg Med 2003;24(3):351–2.

[47] Centers for Disease Control and Prevention. Recommendations for using smallpox vaccine in a pre-event vaccination program. Supplemental recommendations of the Advisory Committee on Immunization Practices (ACIP) and the Healthcare Infection Control Practices Advisory Committee (HICPAC). MMWR Recomm Rep 2003;52(RR-7):1–16.

[48] Centers for Disease Control and Prevention. Vaccinia (smallpox) vaccine: recommendations of the Advisory Committee on Immunization Practices (ACIP), 2001. MMWR Recomm Rep 2001;50(RR-10):1–25.

[49] Borio L, Inglesby T, Peters CJ, et al. Hemorrhagic fever viruses as biological weapons. JAMA 2002;287(18):2391–405.

[50] Centers for Disease Control and Prevention. Management of patients with suspected viral hemorrhagic fever. MMWR Morb Mortal Wkly Rep 1995;44(25):475–9.

[51] Arnon SS, Schechter R, Inglesby TV, et al. Botulinum toxin as a biological weapon. JAMA 2001;285(8):1059–70.

[52] Shapiro RL, Hatheway C, Becher J, et al. Botulism surveillance and emergency response. JAMA 1997;278(5):433–5.

[53] Arnon SS, Schechter R, Maslanka SE, et al. Human botulism immune globulin for the treatment of infant botulism. N Engl J Med 2006;354(5):462–71.

[54] Dennis DT, Inglesby TV, Henderson DA, et al. Tularemia as a biological weapon: medical and public health management. JAMA 2001;285(21):2763–73.

[55] Sato T, Fujita H, Ohara Y, et al. Microagglutination test for early and specific serodiagnosis of tularemia. J Clin Microbiol 1990;28(10):2372–4.

[56] Bevanger L, Macland JA, Naess AI. Agglutinins and antibodies to Francisella tularensis outer membrane antigens in the early diagnosis of disease during an outbreak of tularemia. J Clin Microbiol 1988;26(3):433–7.

[57] Russell P, Eley SM, Fulop MJ, et al. The efficacy of ciprofloxacin and doxycycline against tularemia. J Antimicrob Chemother 1998;41(1):461–5.

[58] Dupont HT, Raoult D, Brouqui P, et al. Epidemiologic features and clinical presentation of acute Q fever in hospitalized patients: 323 French cases. Am J Med 1992;93(4): 427–34.

[59] Millar JK. The chest film findings in Q fever—a series of 35 cases. Clin Radiol 1978;329(4): 371–5.

[60] Raoult D. Treatment of Q fever. Antimicrob Agents Chemother 1993;37(9):1733–6.

[61] Franz DR, Jahrling PB, Friedlander AM, et al. Clinical recognition and management of patients exposed to biological warfare agents. JAMA 1997;278(5):399–411.

[62] Young EJ. Overview of brucellosis. Clin Infect Dis 1995;21(2):283–9.

[63] Barham WB, Church P, Brown JE, et al. Misidentification of Brucella species with use of rapid bacterial identification systems. Clin Infect Dis 1993;17(6):1068–9.

[64] Kaufmann AF, Meltzer MI, Schmid GP. The economic impact of a bioterrorist attack: are prevention and postattack intervention programs justifiable? Emerg Infect Dis 1997;3(2): 83–94.

[65] Centers for Disease Control and Prevention. Laboratory-acquired human glanders—Maryland, May 2000. MMWR Morb Mortal Wkly Rep 2000;49(24):532–5.

[66] Srinivasan A, Kraus CN, DeShazer D, et al. Glanders in a military research microbiologist. N Engl J Med 2001;345(4):256–8.

[67] Mobley JA. Biological warfare in the twentieth century: lessons from the past, challenges for the future. Mil Med 1995;160(11):547–53.

[68] Bauernfeind A, Roller C, Meyer D, et al. Molecular procedure for rapid detection of Burkholderia mallei and Burkholderia pseudomallei. J Clin Microbiol 1998;36(9):2737–41.

[69] Heine HS, England MJ, Waag DM, et al. In vitro antibiotic susceptibilities of Burkholderia mallei (causative agent of glanders) determined by broth microdilution and E-test. Antimicrob Agents Chemother 2001;45(7):2119–21.

[70] Deresiewicz RL, Thaler SJ, Hsu L, et al. Clinical and neurologic manifestations of eastern equine encephalitis. N Engl J Med 1997;336(26):1867–74.

[71] Calisher CH, El-Kafrawi AO, Al-Deen Mahmud MI, et al. Complex-specific immunoglobulin M antibody patterns in humans infected with alphaviruses. J Clin Microbiol 1986;23(1): 155–9.

[72] Ricin. In: Woods JB, editor. Medical management of biological casualties handbook. 6th edition. Fort Detrick (MD): USAMRIID; 2005. p. 93–6.

[73] Challoner KR, McCarron MM. Castor bean intoxication. Ann Emerg Med 1990;19(10): 1177–83.

[74] Leith AG, Griffiths GD, Green MA. Quantification of ricin toxin using a highly sensitive avidin/biotin enzyme-linked immunosorbent assay. J Forensic Sci Soc 1988;28(4):227–36.

[75] Smallshaw JE, Richardson JA, Vitetta ES. RiVax, a recombinant ricin subunit vaccine, protects mice against ricin delivered by gavage or aerosol. Vaccine 2007;25(42):7459–69.

[76] Lorber B. Gas gangrene and other clostridium-associated diseases. In: Mandell GL, Bennett JE, Dolin R, editors. Principles and practice of infectious diseases. 5th edition. Philadelphia: Churchill Livingstone; 2000. p. 2549–61.

[77] Kolavic SA, Kimura A, Simons SL, et al. An outbreak of Shigella dysenteriae type 2 among laboratory workers due to intentional food contamination. JAMA 1997;278(5):396–8.

[78] Torok TJ, Tauxe RV, Wise RP, et al. A large community outbreak of salmonellosis caused by intentional contamination of restaurant salad bars. JAMA 1997;278(5):389–95.

[79] Centers for Disease Control and Prevention. Emerging infectious diseases: outbreak of Salmonella enteritidis associated with nationally distributed ice cream products—Minnesota, South Dakota, and Wisconsin, 1994. MMWR Morb Mortal Wkly Rep 1994; 43(40):740–1.

[80] Centers for Disease Control and Prevention. Multistate outbreak of listeriosis—United States, 2000. MMWR Morb Mortal Wkly Rep 2000;49(50):1129–30.

[81] Centers for Disease Control and Prevention. Diagnosis and management of foodborne illnesses: a primer for physicians. MMWR Recomm Rep 2001;50(RR02):1–69.

[82] Mac Kenzie WR, Hoxie NJ, Proctor ME, et al. A massive outbreak in Milwaukee of cryptosporidium infection transmitted through the public water supply. N Engl J Med 1994; 331(3):161–7.

[83] Talan DA, Moran GJ, Newdow M, et al, for the EMERGEncy ID Net Study Group. Etiology of bloody diarrhea among patients presenting to U.S. emergency departments: prevalence of E. coli O157:H7 and other enteropathogens. Clin Infect Dis 2001;32(4):573–80.

[84] Mead PS, Griffin PM. Escherichia coli O157:H7. Lancet 1998;352(9135):1207–12.

[85] Centers for Disease Control and Prevention. Update: outbreak of Nipah virus, Malyasia and Singapore, 1999. MMWR Morb Mortal Wkly Rep 1999;48(16):335–7.

[86] Daniels P, Ksiazek T, Eaton BT. Laboratory diagnosis of Nipah and Hendra virus infections. Microbes Infect 2001;3(4):289–95.

[87] Chua KB, Lam SK, Goh KJ, et al. The presence of Nipah virus in respiratory secretions and urine of patients during an outbreak of Nipah virus encephalitis in Malaysia. J Infect 2001; 42(1):40–3.

[88] Chong HT, Kamarulzaman A, Tan CT, et al. Treatment of acute Nipah encephalitis with ribavirin. Ann Neurol 2001;49(6):810–3.

[89] Nichol ST, Spiropoulou CF, Morzunov S, et al. Genetic identification of a hantavirus associated with an outbreak of acute respiratory illness. Science 1993;262(5135):914–7.

[90] Duchin JS, Koster F, Peters CJ, et al. Hantavirus pulmonary syndrome: a clinical description of 17 patients with a newly recognized disease. N Engl J Med 1994;330(14):949–55.

[91] Koraka P, Avsic-Zupanc T, Osterhaus AD, et al. Evaluation of two commercially available immunoassays for the detection of hantavirus antibodies in serum samples. J Clin Virol 2000; 17(3):189–96.

[92] Padula PJ, Edelstein A, Miguel SD, et al. Hantavirus pulmonary syndrome outbreak in Argentina: molecular evidence for person-to-person transmission of Andes virus. Virology 1998;241(2):323–30.

[93] Wells RM, Sosa Estani S, Yadon ZE, et al. An unusual hantavirus outbreak in southern Argentina: person-to-person transmission? Emerg Infect Dis 1997;3(2):171–4.

[94] Fabbri M, Maslow MJ. Hantavirus pulmonary syndrome in the United States. Curr Infect Dis Rep 2001;3(3):258–65.

[95] Monath TP. Yellow fever: a medically neglected disease. Rev Infect Dis 1987;9(1):165–75.

[96] Tsai TF. Flaviviruses. In: Mandell GL, Bennett JE, Dolin R, editors. Principles and practice of infectious diseases. 5th edition. Philadelphia: Churchill Livingstone; 2000. p. 1714–36.

[97] Small PM, Fujiwara PI. Management of tuberculosis in the United States. N Engl J Med 2001;345(3):189–210.

ELSEVIER
SAUNDERS

Infect Dis Clin N Am 22 (2008) 189–193

INFECTIOUS
DISEASE CLINICS
OF NORTH AMERICA

Index

Note: Page numbers of article titles are in **boldface** type.

0891-5520/08/$ - see front matter © 2008 Elsevier Inc. All rights reserved.
doi:10.1016/S0891-5520(08)00011-1

id.theclinics.com